NREMT Study Guide 2022-2023

480 Test Questions and Detailed Answer Explanations for the EMT Cognitive Exam (National Registry of Emergency Medical Technicians)

Table of Contents

Introduction

Emergency medical technicians (EMTs) are the connection between an emergency setting and an emergency room (ER). EMTs act as middlemen and provide emergency care to patients outside a hospital setting. They stabilize patients, provide emergency medical services, then transport patients to the appropriate facility. In the United States, EMTs are second in the ranking of emergency service providers:

- EMRs (emergency medical responders)
- EMTs (emergency medical technicians)
- AEMTs (advanced emergency medical technicians)
- Paramedics

Functions of an EMT

First-line response
EMTs offer a first-line response to critical/emergent patients. They respond to 911 calls and attend to patients outside the hospital setting in homes, offices, schools, natural disasters, and so on.

Assessment
On arrival, EMTs quickly assess a patient's clinical status and vital signs, like heart rate, respiratory rate, consciousness, blood pressure, and breathing pattern. They obtain a quick clinical history from surrounding witnesses and determine the best approach to resuscitation.

Resuscitation
EMTs are trained to provide resuscitation where appropriate by stabilizing patients' airways, circulation, and breathing. Apart from resuscitation, EMTs stabilize patients and prepare them for transportation and transfer.

Transportation
Unlike EMRs, who provide only resuscitation services, EMTs are trained to transport patients and transfer them to the appropriate personnel in emergency centers.

Collaboration
EMTs collaborate with members of the emergency team (doctors and nurses) and share information on assessment, clinical features, and interventions that were performed before presentation to the ER.

Education Requirements

High school diploma or GED

Basic education requirements include a high school diploma or a GED. People who do not have a high school diploma can take the GED.

CPR certification

After obtaining a basic education degree, all candidates are expected to earn a certification in cardiopulmonary resuscitation (CPR) in order to qualify for EMT training. Certifications can be obtained from either the American Heart Association or the American Red Cross.

EMT training program

Formal training is needed for certification. This training can be either a diploma or a certificate. These training programs are provided by technical or trade schools, community colleges, and facilities dedicated solely to training people in emergency care.

Accreditation of EMT programs is done by the Commission on Accreditation of Allied Health Education Programs (CAAHEP). Certificate programs provide training in basic skills and procedures for life support, and classes can be a hybrid mixture of on-site, off-site, and fieldwork activities. Certificate and diploma programs take about one to two years to complete. A lot of schools offer flexible options to suit students who work full time.

Associate degrees

EMTs who wish to further their training and become paramedics require an associate's degree after obtaining a Basic EMT certification. Because paramedics provide more comprehensive care than basic EMTs, they receive extensive training on emergency care, airway stabilization, circulation, drugs, patient stabilization, trauma, pharmacology, care of special groups, and more.

EMT certification

EMT certification is provided by the National Registry of Emergency Medical Technicians (NREMT). Candidates are expected to pass the NREMT psychomotor and cognitive tests, after which they are awarded the NREMT certification. That certification is valid for two years. Details of the NREMT will be discussed in full in this book. It is important to note that while most states accept the NREMT certification, some states require state-specific certification.

Career Options

In hospital settings

In hospital settings, EMTs work with emergency units, high-dependency units, intensive care centers, and trauma centers.

Off-hospital settings

EMTs can work in fire departments, police units, disaster units, schools, correctional facilities, private companies, and more.

Career Advancement

EMTs can advance in their careers by upskilling and gaining additional work experience. Alternative EMT career options include:

Emergency room technician

The job descriptions of an emergency medical technician and an emergency room technician are somewhat similar, but unlike EMTs, emergency room technicians work specifically in emergency rooms and clinical facilities.

Registered nurse

EMTs can upskill to become registered nurses and provide nursing and clinical care to patients. Registered nurses are key members of the health team. A career as a registered nurse is flexible and rewarding, with plenty of room for specializing in diverse nursing fields.

Certified phlebotomist

Phlebotomists collect, prepare, and transport blood and other samples to the lab for investigation and diagnosis.

Physician assistant

Physician assistants bridge the gap created by insufficient primary care providers in the United States. They examine, diagnose, and manage patients under a physician's supervision.

Surgical technologist

A surgical technologist is a member of the surgical team who prepares surgical instruments and equipment, disinfects work surfaces and surgical theaters before and after surgeries, and is in charge of surgical supplies. Surgical technologists also assist surgeons by handing them surgical instruments during operations.

Emergency dispatcher
EMTs who want a step down from the stress of emergency care can become emergency dispatchers. Dispatchers receive emergency calls and route them to the appropriate emergency personnel after obtaining all the necessary information from callers.

Health-information technician
EMTs who wish to switch to administrative health care can become health-information technicians, who organize, store, and review patients' medical information.

Offshore medic
Offshore medics provide emergency care to oil rig workers. The job pays well paid but can be stressful, as most people work 12-hour shifts every two weeks.

Radiologic technician
Radiologic technicians maintain radiologic equipment, adjust and operate radiologic equipment, prepare patients, and assess radiologic images.

EMTs can switch careers for any of these reasons:

1. Better pay – Although most EMTs earn a good salary, they can switch to other careers with better pay. For example, registered nurses, nurse practitioners, and physician assistants earn about two to three times more than EMTs.
2. Regular hours – EMTs can switch to careers with regular hours. For example, registered nurses have more regular hours than EMTs.
3. Hazards – Some EMTs switch to careers with reduced physical, biological, and psychological hazards, such as health-care administration.

Pay

The average salary of an EMT is $33,380, with a range of about $21,880 to $56,990. pay depends on these factors:

Location
The states with the highest salaries for EMTs include Maryland ($41,940), Connecticut ($47,360), Alaska ($50,500), and Washington ($76,040). However, EMTs must consider the impact of housing, food, and transportation before considering pay based on location.

Employer
The following industries offer the highest EMT salaries: ambulances ($30,800), hospitals ($35,990), and local governments ($35,620).

Work experience

Advanced EMTs and paramedics can earn as high as $56,990 per year. These people make up 10% of top EMT earners in the United States.

Traits of a Successful EMT

Endurance

A successful EMT can withstand physical stress from pushing, pulling, and lifting patients. EMTs also require psychological stamina because they are regularly exposed to patients who have suffered from trauma, accidents, etc.

Critical thinking

EMTs must think critically and make quick decisions in high-pressure environments. EMTs with these abilities save the lives patients who need acute resuscitation.

Collaboration and teamwork

EMTs should be able to work with their colleagues and other members of the health team. Collaboration involves communicating, receiving and giving feedback, and exchanging other types of information.

Communication skills

EMTs should be able to use therapeutic communication techniques with their patients. These techniques help establish trust, collaboration, and patient-health personnel relationships.

Pros and Cons of Becoming an EMT

Pros

1. Job satisfaction – The job is a satisfying one because an EMT can see immediate effects when they resuscitate and stabilize patients. For example, a patient with central cyanosis and respiratory distress can benefit immediately from oxygen supplementation.
2. Career alternatives – An EMT can switch to other health career alternatives whenever the need arises. Such flexibility in alternate career pathways makes being an EMT a versatile career.

Cons

1. Burnout – Repeated physical and psychological stress can cause burnout. EMTs who repeatedly witness trauma and disasters are at risk of developing anxiety disorders, post-traumatic stress disorder, and more.
2. Hazards – Like other health workers, EMTs are exposed to physical hazards from pushing, pulling, lifting, straining, etc. They are also exposed to biological hazards from blood, blood products, and bodily fluids, as well as psychological hazards from working in high-pressure environments.
3. Pay – The salary for an EMT is low compared to other health workers like registered nurses, phlebotomists, physician assistants, technologists, and others.

Differences between a Paramedic and an EMT

Education requirements

Paramedics require extensive training in resuscitation, stabilization, and transport. While formal training in EMS may not be required for EMTs, an associate's degree is required for anyone who chooses to become a paramedic. Paramedics must also pass the national registry exams for both EMTs and paramedics.

Scope of practice

A paramedic has more job responsibilities than an EMT. The scope of practice includes basic skills required for EMTs and advanced skills in resuscitation, stabilization, and transport.

Chapter 1: The NREMT Exam

The National Registry Emergency Medical Technician Exam (NREMT) is a licensing exam used in certifying emergency medical technicians in the United States and Canada. This exam is created and administered by the National Registry, an NGO that offers certification exams to professionals who offer emergency medical services. The National Registry also offers certifications in Emergency Medical Responder (NREMR), Paramedics (NRP), and Advanced Emergency Medical Technician (NRAEMT).

For over 50 years, the National Registry has been committed to certifying EMS providers who can guarantee the safety of the public. To do this, the National Registry uses a set of formulated and standardized cognitive and task-oriented skills that can verify the proficiency of EMS providers in the United States, the District of Columbia, and all US territories.

The National Registry also provides resources for ongoing and continuous learning, improves employer-employee relationships via employer resources and programs, and provides other resources. The National Registry prides itself on its ability to provide services that are diverse, nondiscriminatory, and inclusive.

The NREMT exams provided by the National Registry are accredited by the National Commission for Certifying Agencies (NCCA). This board is the sole accreditor for certifying EMS professionals. The accreditation provided by the NCCA means that the National Registry has met all the requirements in developing, implementing, and maintaining certification exams.

Eligibility Requirements

1. Education

You are expected to have completed an EMT program that is accredited by both the state and the appropriate accreditation board. This course should be completed two years before you apply for the NREMT Exam.

2. BLS Certification

You are expected to have a current CPR-BLS certification.

How to Register for the NREMT Exam

1. Application

Application is done solely online on www.nremt.org.
You can apply to take the NREMT by following these steps:

Create a profile – This stage is required for new users. Previous users can log in using their usernames and passwords. Remember to use a valid email address.
Fill out the application form – You must ensure that you meet the requirements for eligibility by filling in the required information as instructed.

2. Review

The registry will confirm the details of your application form. Confirmation of the education program is done by the program director. If you submit an incomplete or erroneous application, you will be contacted for correction.

3. Authorization to test

Once you have completed your application, paid the required application fees, and had application forms verified by your program director, you will receive authorization to test (ATT) within one to two working days. This processing time can take longer.

Note that you will not receive ATT notification via email. Instead, you will get a notification in your dashboard on the website at the Application Status taskbar. You can view and print your ATT and read instructions on how to schedule your exams via Pearson VUE. The ATT is valid for only 90 days from the time it is uploaded on your dashboard. It cannot be extended once it expires. If your ATT expires, you must pay a new application fee and complete a new application.

4. Scheduling an exam

To schedule an exam, read the instructions on the ATT. Scheduling is done on the PSI website. On the PSI website, first-time exam takers are required to create an account on the website and use the ID number provided in their notification.

After you schedule the exam, Pearson VUE will send a notification email that confirms the scheduled test date and time, including phone numbers and address of the test center and directions to the test venue. Reservations are made on a first-come, first-served basis. Exams may be scheduled any day Monday through Saturday except holidays. Allow at least four business days between the day you receive your eligibility letter and your preferred test date.

5. Rescheduling/canceling the exam

You must reschedule your exam within the 90-day ATT window. Exams should be rescheduled at least one business day before the test date. You will be charged $25 for canceling/rescheduling. Rescheduling fees will not be refunded if you end up taking the exam on the original date.

All rescheduling must be done via the Pearson VUE website. Failure to do so leads to automatic cancellation of the exam. You must then reapply and pay new application fees.

Reschedules must be done promptly because seating arrangements are given on a first-come, first-served basis. Failure to reschedule will lead to the automatic cancellation of the exam. There are no refunds for the exam if you do not reschedule or cancel a test appointment. Refunds are also not given if a request to opt out of the exam is made after the 90-day window has expired. Refunds are given only to candidates who are within the 90-day window and have never made a scheduling appointment with PSI.

6. No-show policy

If you fail to reschedule your exam at least 24 hours before the test date and fail to show up for the test, you will receive a "no-show" status on your dashboard. No refunds will be given unless there is sufficient evidence to warrant it. Appeals can be made and are reviewed on a case-by-case basis.

Application Fees

The NREMT application fee is $80. You can pay via check or credit card (MasterCard, American Express and Visa only). Split payments and debit cards are not accepted. Payments must be made in US dollars online. Payment via fax or mail is not accepted.

Additional fees

Paper applications for recertification cost an additional $5. Returned checks require an additional $35 fee. All outstanding payments should be made within 10 working days of notification.

Refunds

You will receive a refund if you cancel your exam within your ATT period or incorrectly fill out an application form. Refunds will not be given after 90 days. Refunds are made in the same format in which payment was made.

Retake Policies

You have six attempts at the NREMT exam. If you are unsuccessful at the third attempt, you must complete a remedial program before attempting the test again. You will be required to show proof of completion of the remedial program. Requirements for remedial programs vary from state to state.

Option 1 – States under the NCCP require 20 hours of the EMT National Competency Component.
Option 2 – States using the traditional model require 24 completed hours of the EMT refresher course.
Option 3 – Completion of 20-hour or 24-hour remedial programs from any suitable and accredited education program from vocational schools, online sources, community colleges, EMS agencies and others.

To retest, you are required to wait at least 15 days after the previous test date. You must start a new application process and pay a new application fee.

Recertification

Recertification is required every two years. Recertification can be done via either a recertification exam or continuing education.

Recertification by exam
Professionals who use this method are expected to take a cognitive NREMT exam. They are given one attempt to pass the exam one year before the expiration of their current license. Once they pass, they can upload their exam forms, along with other required documents, for recertification.

Recertification by continuing education
The NCCP requires 40 hours of continuing education by national component, individual component, and local component.

A total of 20 hours is required in the national component. Professionals can provide proof of 7 hours of education in these fields: airway and respiration (1.5 hours), cardiovascular (6 hours), trauma (1.5 hours), medical (6 hours) and operations (5 hours). A total of 10 hours is required in the local component.

A total of 10 hours is required for the individual component. The maximum required hours is 10. Materials for continuing education may be accredited by the CAPCE or state.

What to Expect on Exam Day

1. Check-in

You should arrive at your designated testing center at least 30 minutes before your scheduled exam time. This is to enable you to verify your identity during recheck, identify your seat, and be comfortably settled before the exam begins. If you arrive more than 15 minutes after the exam begins, you will not be allowed to take the exam.

Items that are prohibited from the testing center include reference materials, like books, papers, and dictionaries; and personal items, like purses, headwear, hoodies, veils, coats, and briefcases. Pearson and the National Registry will not take responsibility for any missing or stolen items, so these items should be left at home or in a vehicle.

2. Identification

You must present two forms of identification (ID). The primary identification should have your full name, photo, and signature. Accepted forms of ID are passports, green cards, driver's licenses, state identification cards, national identity cards, and permanent resident cards. Your ID must have your name and signature. Examples are Social Security cards, credit cards, employment cards, and student cards. Temporary ID is not acceptable.

If your name in the eligibility letter differs from the one on your ID, you must show proof of name change (a court order, divorce papers, or marriage license). If you do not have an approved ID, you will not be allowed to take the exam. You will be noted as having missed the testing appointment, and no refunds will be made.

Before the exam begins, you are expected to confirm your name and the nature of the exam. You also must agree to the rules and regulations of PSI and the National Registry.

Mode of Exam Delivery

The NREMT exams are CBT exams administered via a testing facility. A test administrator will assign you to a seat and computer. Before the exam begins, an untimed practice test is done to familiarize users with the exam's software interface. After this, you must assent to a nondisclosure agreement before commencing the exam.

For security, you are expected to show your approved primary and secondary identity cards before testing. These cards will be verified by a security system. Also, you will be asked to sign to show attendance and have your photo taken. Video and audio recordings of the exam will be made.

Exam length

The NREMT exam lasts for two hours. It has 70 to 120 multiple-choice questions. Ten test items are unscored. You will be unable to differentiate a scored item from an unscored item.

Exam breaks

Test breaks are not allowed during the exam. You are expected to attempt all questions.

Testing Accommodations

If you require testing accommodations, you must fill out the Test Accommodations Form from the website. All forms requesting accommodations must be signed by the appropriate health-care professional. The National Registry will assess your request based on the information in the form and provide accommodations as needed.

Rules and Regulations

Testing facilities

1. You are not allowed to discuss or communicate with other test-takers in any fashion after entering the examination hall.
2. You are not permitted to copy, duplicate, communicate, or transmit the test content for any reason. Copying and duplicating test content is a violation of the PSI's security policy. If you violate this rule, you are at risk of being disqualified from the exam and will be reported to the National Registry and security officials.
3. Electronic devices of any kind are banned from the exam hall.
4. Personal items and effects are banned from the exam hall. These items should be stored in a safe place before admission into the hall. PSI is not liable for any missing or stolen property.
5. Abusive behavior toward the testing center staff is prohibited. You are expected to be courteous, professional, and respectful of both the staff and the rules and regulations of the exam. If you are abusive to the staff, you are at risk of forfeiting the exam and will be reported to the National Registry and security personnel.
6. Third parties are prohibited from entering the examination room.
7. You are prohibited from leaving the building or using telephones during the examination.
8. You are not allowed breaks during the exam.

How the Exam Is Developed

The NREMT exam is a CAT exam. This means that the number of test items and their difficulty differs by candidate. However, all test scores are weighted by a passing standard. Pass/fail status is determined by your ability to prove entry-level competency. In the CAT, you are given questions based on previous answers. For example, if you answer questions correctly, you are given more difficult questions. If you answer these questions correctly, you are taken to another category.

Practice analysis

Research is done on current principles and practices in the core domains of EMS. Data is collected from EMS professionals, employers, and educators. After collation, the data is analyzed and results are used as a guide in creating test items.

Item writers

Experts in EMS are hired as members of the examination committee. These experts are from diverse geographical, practice, and demographic regions in the United States. Experts are also hired based on clinical experience, qualifications, and skills. They are then trained in the principles of writing EMS test questions.

Reviewers

Reviewers are professionals who assess test items for reliability, discrimination level, difficulty, and performance.

Content teams

This includes professionals in EMS. The president of the National Registry selects members of content teams. Members of content teams are responsible for creating and updating competent statements and test outlines, reviewing data from completed exams, evaluating test items created by item writers, approving the exam forms used on the test day, and reviewing items in item banks.

How Exams Are Scored

The NREMT's passing standard is based on a set of criteria created by the Board of Directors of the National Registry and is revised every three years. The Angoff Method is used to analyze test scores. In this analysis, test items are scored and evaluated based on the relationship between the ability of the candidate and the test answered. This means that test items with a high difficulty have high scores. However, pass/fail is awarded based on the total number of correctly answered questions. When a candidate answers a question correctly, the person's ability score increases. If they answer a question incorrectly, their ability score decreases.

Equating is used to scale down test results because candidates are given tests in different forms. This means that candidates who answer a higher number of difficult questions will need to answer fewer questions, and candidates who answer a lower number of difficult questions will need to answer more questions. Word descriptors like *above passing*, *below passing*, and *near passing* are used to describe pass/fail status.

Getting Test Results

Results will be posted to your dashboard two working days after you take the exam. If you do not see your results after five working days, you should contact the registry. Results are not sent by email, fax, or telephone.

Candidates' Performance Reports

Performance reports are not available to successful candidates. Performance reports act as a guide for unsuccessful candidates to help them objectively assess their strengths and weaknesses. This helps candidates focus their studying before retesting.

The performance of candidates in each content category is described as:

Above passing

This means that a candidate has good knowledge of this content category. This does not rule out future reviews before retesting.

Near passing

A candidate's performance was a little below/above the passing standard.

Below passing

A candidate requires more review in this content category.

Please note that pass/fail status is awarded based on overall performance and not on individual performance in each content category.

Exam Review

You can request a review of your test scores. However, you can request a review of only specific test items. These items will be reviewed according to their accuracy, relevance to the scope of practice, and impact on the overall test score. A review is not done on the passing standard or examination items.

If you wish to review certain test items, send your request within a month of receipt of your results. A rescoring fee of $150 is required. After the payment is confirmed, a new score report will be sent within 30 days of payment. If the review process reveals irregularities on the first score report, you will be refunded the rescoring fee.

Tips on How to Pass the NREMT Exam

Passing the NREMT exams requires a combination of preparation, organization, and mental attitude. Adequate preparation has a lot to do with the type of resource materials you prepare with, the amount of time you spend preparing, and your capacity for recall.

How to choose the right resource material

Here are a few things to consider before choosing the right study material for your exams:

1. Relevance – Your study material should be relevant to the exam. To increase your chances of selecting relevant study material, buy resources that your tutors, colleagues, and peers recommend.
2. Current – How current is your study material? The National Registry reviews the NREMT exams every three years; therefore, your study material should be current, updated, and revised to reflect the standard.
3. Cost – Beware of outrageously expensive study materials. There are reasonably priced study guides available.
4. Highlights – Your study material should give highlights on the distribution of test questions and priority areas to focus on. The right study material should help you narrow your reading to specific and key areas.
5. Comprehensive rationale – Your study material should give a comprehensive rationale for all test questions and answers. This fine-tunes your critical thinking and helps you identify subtle words and distinctions you might not have otherwise noticed.

6. Organization – Your study material should be organized methodically. Study materials that break down complex material into outlines and sections improve your recall.

How much time should you spend studying?

There is no one-size-fits-all study duration, but there are a few basic factors that can help you choose the best study schedule for your needs.

1. Start early – Early preparation increases your chances of success because you have time to prepare and make mistakes. Yes, you can make mistakes in your studying, especially if you are taking the exam for the first time. You can start with the wrong resource material or have an inefficient study plan. Whatever the error, early preparation allows you room to revise and adjust your study plan as needed.
2. Have a study goal – Remember, your study goal must be SMART: Specific, Measurable, Achievable, Relevant, and Time-Bound. For example, let's say you have a study goal to review 400 study guide questions in a month. This goal has met three requirements of the SMART goal. It is specific, measurable, and time-bound. You now have to assess whether that goal is attainable. To do so, you will have to determine how many questions you can answer in a day, how much time will be allotted to each study session, and whether the amount of time allocated is feasible.
3. Create a study timetable – A study plan helps you track your progress and keeps you disciplined and focused. For example, let's say you have assessed the feasibility of reviewing 400 questions in one month. Your next step will be to create a detailed study timetable that shows how much time is allocated to each study session.
4. Choose a suitable study method – Group studying has its advantages and disadvantages, and so does studying solo. Some candidates study efficiently on their own, while others do better in groups. A good tip is to use both forms of study, devoting more time to the one you prefer. That way, you can harness the benefits of both.
5. Participate in extracurricular activities – You should factor rest, sleep, breaks, and physical activity into your study timetable.

How to improve your recall

Recall is an important aspect of studying. After all, what is the point of studying if you cannot recall significant information when you need to? Here are a few tips to improve your recall:

1. Read actively – As much as possible, try to engage your mind in the text you are reading. Here are a few tips to help you read actively:
    A. Read with a focus – By giving you areas to focus on, study materials increase your engagement and concentration.
    B. Take notes as you read – As you read, make notes, create mnemonics, create questions, or create a post-reading to-do list. You can also highlight sections of the text that you want to revisit.
    C. Take breaks – Active reading requires focus and effort. For this reason, study sessions should be kept to a range of two to three hours. Anything longer, and you may struggle to concentrate.
2. Study in a group – Group study is an effective form of active reading.
3. Use mnemonics – Mnemonics are great tools for improving your recall. However, use them only after you understand the concepts you are studying. Mnemonics include but are not limited to acronyms, rhymes, imagery, chunking, and the use of loci.
4. Understand first principles – Understanding topics from a first-principles basis improves your ability to store and retrieve information. When studying, always try to link the information together, methodically building on your knowledge.
5. Sleep – Sleep consolidates short-term memory. An adult requires an average of seven to nine hours of sleep a night. Therefore, when you create your study plan, factor in your need to get adequate sleep.

How to be organized

To increase your chances of success, you should organize your activities before and during the exam.

1. Early registration – We discussed the importance of early registration in the previous chapter. Early registration increases your chances of success because it switches you into study mode. Early registration also gives you room to mitigate the effects of unforeseen circumstances.
2. Punctuality – You should show up early to your exam center. Always aim to show up at least 30 minutes before test time. This gives you a chance to verify your identity, acquaint yourself with the rules of the examination, and adjust to the environment.
3. Dressing – Dress comfortably and professionally for the exam. Coats are not allowed into the exam hall. If you get cold easily, do not wear clothes made with thin fabric.

Having the right mental attitude

A positive mental attitude is important for taking the exam, particularly if you are retaking the test. Here are a few tips to boost your mental attitude.

1. Study group peers – You can get support from your study group peers who share your goal.
2. Tutors and mentors – You can also get support and encouragement from your tutors and mentors.
3. Successful candidates – People who have successfully passed the test can give you good advice.
4. Visualization and affirmation – These tools can boost your confidence and improve your attitude toward the exam.
5. Sleep – Adequate rest can improve your mood, attitude, and cognitive functions.

Chapter 2: Content Overview

Airway, Ventilation, and Respiration

This section makes up 18% to 22% of test content. Topic areas include:

Anatomy of the respiratory system

The upper airway
The upper airway is made up of the nasal cavity, the pharynx, and the larynx. During inspiration, air goes from the nose into the nasal cavity. In the nasal cavity, the air is humidified and dust particles are filtered by nasal hairs. Humidified air currents move into the pharynx, then into the larynx. The entrance of the larynx is guarded by the epiglottis, which prevents the passage of food into the lower respiratory tract.

The lower airway
The lower airway is made up of the trachea and bronchi. Air flows from the trachea into the carina, then into the main bronchi. From the main bronchi, it moves into the alveoli in the bronchioles, which are highly vascularized tissues that allow the exchange of oxygen for carbon dioxide.

The lungs are protected by the rib cage. Below the lungs is the diaphragm, a fibromuscular structure that separates the lungs from the abdominal organs. The diaphragm is also an accessory muscle for inspiration. It is controlled by the autonomic branch of the nervous system.

The lungs are further protected by the pleura, a fibrous sac that encloses the lungs. The inner layer of the pleura is called the visceral pleura; it lubricates the lungs and reduces friction. It also provides nutrients and oxygen to the lungs. The outer layer is called the parietal pleura. It is tough and fibrous and protects the lungs from injury.

Physiology of the respiratory system

During inspiration, the diaphragm increases intrathoracic pressure by becoming flat and pulling the ribs outward and upward. The lungs expand, and air flows into the nasal cavity and down to the alveoli in the bronchioles.

The alveoli are made up predominantly of Type 1 pneumocytes, which are squamous cells that allow the exchange of carbon dioxide for oxygen. During exhalation, the diaphragm shortens back to its initial length. This causes the chest cavity to return to its original size and allows the expulsion of air through the nose.

Oxygen in the alveolar capillaries is carried via the hemoglobin in red blood cells into the systemic circulation. At tissue spaces, oxygen is uncoupled from hemoglobin and diffuses into the cells. Carbon dioxide diffuses from the tissue into the capillaries and venous circulation.

Factors that control respiratory rate

The autonomic system in the pons and medulla controls breathing. Factors that control respiratory rate include:

Serum carbon dioxide – Hypercapnia triggers the chemoreceptors in the brain.
pH – Low blood pH and acidosis trigger the chemoreceptors in the brain and stimulate respiration.

Voluntary inspiration and expiration are controlled via the motor neurons in the cerebral cortex. The functions of these neurons can be overridden by chemoreceptors in the respiratory centers in the hindbrain.

How to assess the respiratory system

1. Inspection

Normal respiratory rates:
Infants – 25–50/min
Children – 5–30/min
Adults – 12–20/min

Rhythm – Regular or irregular
Abnormal rhythm – Kussmaul breathing, Biot's breathing, apnea, hyperpnea, Cheyne-Stokes breathing, apneustic breathing, and others.
Signs of respiratory distress – Use of accessory muscles of respiration, pursed lips, flaring of nasal alar, tachypnea, cyanosis, evidence of shock.

2. Palpation

Trachea – Centralization or displacement, tactile fremitus, chest expansion whether equal or unequal.

3. Auscultation

Breath sounds – Present, diminished or absent. Assess whether the tidal volume is normal or shallow.

Special considerations in the anatomy of pediatric patients

Pediatric patients have smaller mouths and nasal cavities. These structures are more prone to obstruction. Also, because the pharynx of infants is smaller, they are prone to obstruction since their tongues occupy more space than adults. Infant tracheas are narrower, softer and more flexible. Their diaphragms are also smaller and softer. Infants are obligate nasal breathers and depend on the diaphragm for breathing.

Features of efficient assisted ventilation

1. The chest is rising and falling at each ventilation.
2. The respiratory rate is about 10–12/min for adults and about 12–20/min for pediatric patients.
3. The heart rate picks up and stabilizes.
4. The skin color improves.

Techniques for opening the airway

Head-tilt and chin-lift

This is used after a cervical injury has been ruled out. To do this, push down on the patient's forehead to tilt the head backward. Support the chin with the pads of your second and third fingers and push the mandible upward. This maneuver opens the pharynx by displacing the tongue.

Jaw thrust

This maneuver is performed on patients with a suspected injury to the cervical spine. The EMS provider stands at the head of the stretcher and lifts the mandible by supporting the temples and the rami of the mandible. The jaw should point upward until the incisors in the lower jaw are higher than those in the upper jaw. Do not put pressure on the soft tissues on the neck while performing this maneuver.

Suctioning equipment

Suction units

This includes mounted suction units, hand-operated suction units, and portable suction units. The manual suction device works without electricity or batteries. The suction created with this equipment is often inconsistent and unpredictable. Because of this, its use has been phased out.

Mounted suction devices are commonly used in ambulances and are easier to use. Portable suction devices are the most versatile. They are battery powered and easily moved because of their size. Since they are battery powered, it is advisable to carry extra batteries.

Suction catheters

Hard suction catheter – This catheter, also called a tonsil tip or tonsil sucker, is hard and rigid. It is used to suction unresponsive patients. It is also used for pediatric patients. During insertion in pediatric patients, the back of the tonsils should not be touched with this catheter.

Soft catheter – This is also called a French catheter. It is used in suctioning the nasopharynx and conscious patients.

How to suction

1. Inspect the suction device before it is used.
2. Switch on the suction unit and assess its function. If there is no measuring gauge, suction the tip of your finger and note traction.
3. Attach the appropriate suction catheter. A hard catheter should be used for unconscious and pediatric patients. A soft catheter should be used for conscious patients.
4. Insert the catheter into the patient's mouth. Do not proceed further than the base of the tongue. Turn on the suction machine. Do not suction for more than 15 seconds at a time. Suction time should be reduced for pediatric patients.
5. Patients with secretions that cannot be easily removed via suctioning should be log rolled; the oropharynx should be cleaned manually.
6. In patients with copious secretions, intervals should be given to assist the patient in ventilation for about two minutes.
7. The catheter and tubing should be rinsed after use to prevent obstruction.

How to perform assisted ventilation

Bag and mask ventilation (BVM)

This can be done by one person or two; however, the two-person technique is preferred because the mask forms a tight seal over the patient's nose and gives adequate ventilation. A nasopharyngeal airway is used to keep the airway patent if there are no contraindications to its use. Oropharyngeal airways are avoided if the patient is conscious with an intact gag reflex. Patients with cervical injury, obesity, short necks, or poor dentition that can affect the sealing of the mask may require a supraglottic airway device unless contraindicated.

Indications

Indications for BVM ventilation include emergency ventilation in patients with respiratory failure, apnea, and inevitable respiratory arrest.

Contraindications

Contraindications include advanced directives such as a do not resuscitate (DNR) order.

Disadvantages

The maximum volume of a BVM is about 1600 mL. This volume is less than that provided by mouth-to-mask. Also, use of a BVM is difficult for single EMT personnel when maintaining an airtight seal. It may require airway devices. It can cause stomach insufflation. If this occurs, an NG tube must be passed to relieve the distension.

Positioning for BVM ventilation

Patients without suspected cervical injury are placed in the sniffing position. Patients with suspected cervical injury are placed in the supine position. The modified jaw thrust is done.

How to do the two-person BVM technique

1. The more experienced person positions the mask over the patient and maintains an adequate seal while the second person squeezes the bag.
2. The person handling the mask stands at the head of the stretcher, while the person handling the bag stands at the side of the bed.
3. The person handling the mask must be sure to avoid putting pressure on the patient's eyes. The nose bridge, malar eminences, and lower lip must be tightly sealed.
4. The traditional method of holding the mask is the C-E grip. After confirming a tight seal, the second person attaches the mask to the bag, and ventilation is commenced.

One-person BVM technique

In this technique, the person handles both the mask and the bag. Most people handle the mask with their nondominant hand while the dominant hand maintains a seal with the mask. For proper sealing, the bridge of the nose, malar eminence, and alveolar ridge of the mandible must be covered properly. The C technique is used to support the mask by forming and maintaining a tight seal around the patient's nose.

Mouth-to-mask BVM ventilation

1. Give 30 chest compressions.
2. Next, ensure the mask is sealed by stabilizing the top of the mask with your fingers with one hand and the bottom part of the mask with the thumb of the other hand.
3. If there is no suspected injury to the cervical spine, open the airway using the head tilt and chin lift.
4. Give one breath in one second and inspect the chest.

Mouth-to-mouth ventilation

This method is used in cases where there is no access to supplemental oxygen or a BVM. Since exhaled air contains 17% oxygen, mouth-to-mouth ventilation is an effective method of giving artificial oxygen. Breaths should not be rapidly or forcefully given. Doing this can cause insufflation of the stomach, vomiting, and aspiration.

1. Open the airway using the head-tilt/chin-lift or modified jaw thrust as indicated.
2. Pinch the patient's nose closed.
3. Put your other hand on the patient's forehead to stabilize yourself, then blow into the patient's mouth for one second. Your lips should form a tight seal around the patient's mouth.
4. Assess the rising of the chest.
5. Give chest compression if the chest does not rise after two breaths.

Airway-assisting devices

Nasopharyngeal airways

Nasopharyngeal airways are flexible tubes used to keep the tongue from obstructing the posterior pharynx. One end of the tube is flared, while the other end is beveled. The beveled end is inserted into the pharynx through the nostril.

Indications

1. Suitable for use in patients with spontaneous respiration and obstruction of the upper part of the airway.
2. Suitable for semiconscious patients with an intact gag reflex.
3. Suitable for use in cases where the oropharyngeal airway cannot be used (such as trismus or trauma to the oral cavity).
4. Useful as an adjunct to BVM ventilation.

Contraindications

An absolute contraindication is a fracture of the cribriform plate.
A relative contraindication is a trauma to the nasal cavity.

Complications

Complications include epistaxis from trauma to the nasal cavity, gagging, vomiting, aspiration pneumonia, and sinusitis.

Equipment needed

Nonsterile gloves, sheets, mask, towels, appropriate-sized nasopharyngeal airways, lubricant and anesthetic gels, suctioning units, Magill forceps, nasogastric tubes, and suction catheters.

Positioning

If there are no suspected injuries to the cervical spine, put the patient in the sniffing position. If there is suspected injury to the spine, use the modified jaw-thrust maneuver.

Procedure

1. First, clear the oropharynx of vomitus, foreign bodies, and secretions.
2. Assess the size of the patient's airway by measuring the nasopharyngeal airway from the tip of the nose to the tragus of the ear. Open each nostril and inspect the size. Choose the nostril with the widest opening.
3. Lubricate the airway with lubricant or anesthetic gel.
4. Inspect the airway posterior to the floor of the nasal septum. The beveled end of the airway should face upward. This prevents the risk of trauma to the septum and consequent epistaxis.
5. Pass the airway under the inferior turbinate.
6. If there is resistance during insertion, rotate the airway and gently advance further.

Oropharyngeal airway

Oropharyngeal airways are rigid airway devices used to displace the tongue from the posterior wall of the pharynx and maintain patency of the pharyngeal airway.

Indications

Oropharyngeal airways are used as assistive devices in BVM. They are also used in unconscious patients with spontaneous breathing, as long as patients have an absent gag reflex.

Contraindications

Absolute contraindications include an active gag reflex in a fully conscious patient. Other relative contraindications include trauma to the oral cavity and spasms of the muscles responsible for chewing (trismus).

Complications

Complications include gagging, vomiting and aspiration, and obstruction of the airway caused by the use of an inappropriate-sized oropharyngeal airway.

Positioning

Place the patient in the sniffing position if no cervical injury is suspected. Patients with suspected injury to the cervical spine should be placed in the supine position and positioned using the jaw-thrust maneuver.

Procedure

1. Remove foreign bodies, vomitus, and oral secretions from the oral cavity and oropharynx.
2. Measure the size of the airway by measuring the airway on the patient's cheek. The tip of the airway should touch the angle of the ramus of the mandible.
3. Insert the airway into the oral cavity. The tip of the airway should face the roof of the mouth.
4. As you get to the posterior part of the oropharynx, rotate the airway 180 degrees to prevent pushing the tongue back into the posterior wall. An alternative is to use a tongue blade to press on the tongue as you advance into the airway. The tip of the blade should point toward the floor of the mouth.
5. When the airway is fully inside the oropharynx, the flange of the device should be at the patient's lips.

Oxygen Delivery Systems

Oxygen cylinders

There are different sizes of oxygen cylinders. They include:

1. D cylinder – 350 L capacity
2. E cylinder – 625 L capacity
3. M cylinder – 3000 L capacity
4. G cylinder – 5300 L capacity
5. H cylinder – 6900 L capacity

Oxygen tanks should be handled with care because they are pressurized. Because oxygen oxidizes, it is combustible. Care must be taken to prevent leakage and explosion.

Although dry oxygen is not dangerous, some respiratory emergencies require intervention with humidified oxygen. Some of these emergencies include smoke inhalation and inhalational burns, croup, asthma, and inhalation of toxins.

How to use the oxygen cylinder

1. First, remove the seal from the gauge.
2. Open the valve, then quickly shut it to burp the cylinder.
3. Couple the regulator-flow meter to the tank.
4. Attach the oxygen-delivery device to the flow meter.
5. Adjust the flow meter to the required setting.

Advantages of oxygen cylinders

Although oxygen cylinders are the least convenient mode of oxygen supply, they are still in demand due to the concentration of oxygen provided.

Disadvantages

Oxygen cylinders are bulky, heavy, and not convenient for ambulatory emergency services.

Oxygen concentrators

Oxygen concentrators are also called oxygen generators. These devices pull oxygen from room air, filtering the oxygen from bacterial dust and other particles until concentrated oxygen of about 90% or more is collected. Oxygen concentrators provide oxygen at a rate of 0.5–5 L/min.

The two types of oxygen concentrators are stationary and portable. Stationary concentrators provide a constant supply of oxygen and are used for long-term oxygen therapy because they save money and are safer. Portable oxygen concentrators are used in ambulatory services and are good for promoting compliance.

Advantages of oxygen concentrators

Oxygen concentrators are easy to use because they do not require refilling. They are run by electricity and supply oxygen on demand.

Portable concentrators are ideal for ambulatory emergency services and transportation. They are cost effective because the cost of maintenance is low compared to oxygen cylinders.

Disadvantages of oxygen concentrators

Oxygen concentrators require electricity to function, and this can be a problem in situations where the electricity supply is cut (such as disasters).

Oxygen-delivery systems

These systems deliver oxygen from oxygen units to the patient. They include low-flow systems and high-flow systems. Low-flow oxygen systems provide oxygen at a rate that is lower than the rate of inspired air, while high-flow oxygen systems provide oxygen at a rate higher than that of inspired air. In this case, the FIO2 is not affected by the rate, depth, and pattern of the patient's breathing.

Low-flow oxygen-delivery systems

Nasal cannulae

Nasal cannulae are the most commonly used oxygen-delivery systems, especially for mild forms of hypoxia. Nasal cannulae give oxygen at a rate of 1–6 L/min. Rate flows that are more than 6 L/min can cause drying of the nasal mucosa. Nasal cannulae are easily dislodged from the nostrils and are unsuitable for use in patients with deviated nasal polyps or septa. They are, however, convenient for use because patients can use them while eating and speaking.

Simple face mask

The simple face mask delivers oxygen at a rate of 5–10 L/min. It is useful in patients with moderate hypoxia. The simple face mask covers the patient's nose and mouth and has exhalation ports at the side, through which carbon dioxide passes. The oxygen delivered via the face mask can be humidified to prevent dryness of the nasal mucosa. Unlike with nasal cannulae, patients cannot eat, drink, or talk with a nasal mask. Also, some patients may feel claustrophobic.

Non-rebreather mask

A non-rebreather mask has a high FiO2. It has a reservoir bed that delivers high oxygen concentrations, a one-way valve that prevents backflow of expired air, and a flow gauge. It can deliver oxygen at 10–15 L/min. This mask is very useful in patients with severe hypoxia. However, side effects include vomiting, aspiration, and carbon dioxide poisoning.

Transtracheal oxygen catheter (TTOC)

This catheter, which delivers oxygen percutaneously into the trachea, is useful in patients with apnea and hypoxemia. This oxygen-delivery system is not popular because of the skill needed to use the catheter. Also, its value in elderly patients with hypoxemia is unclear. The TTOC delivers oxygen at a rate of 0.5–4 L/min.

High-flow oxygen-delivery systems

Rebreather mask

Rebreather masks do not have a one-way valve. Both the expired air and inspired oxygen are collected in a reservoir bag.

Venturi mask

A Venturi mask allows optimum delivery of FIO2 at a rate that is higher than the patient's peak expiratory flow. The mask has a bottle of water; a nebulized, corrugated tube; a mask; and a drainage bag. This mask does not dry out the nasal mucosa, but some patients find it restrictive because it disrupts eating and speaking. It is, however, useful for patients with COPD.

High-flow nasal cannula

This cannula has a nasal cannula, a humidifier, an air-oxygen blender, and a flow generator. It can provide oxygen up to a rate of 60 L/min. The FIO2 and flow rates can be adjusted to suit the patient's needs. These features improve the patient's residual capacity, enhance clearance of the mucous membranes, and reduce the work of breathing.

Common respiratory emergency causes and clinical features

Respiratory arrest

Causes – Causes include decreased respiratory effort, airway obstruction, and weakness of respiratory muscles.

Airway obstruction

Causes – Causes of upper airway obstruction include loss of consciousness and muscle tone, mucus, blood; vomitus, foreign bodies, muscle spasms, edema of the vocal cords, inflammation of the trachea or epiglottis from infection (for example, croup), epiglottitis, trauma, tumors, being less than four months old, and congenital anomalies. Causes of lower airway obstruction include bronchospasm, aspiration, drowning, pneumonia, pulmonary hemorrhage, and pulmonary edema.

Decreased respiratory effort

Causes – Causes include disorders affecting the central nervous system like tumors, strokes, infection, central nervous system disorders that increase intracranial pressure, metabolic disorders like drug overdose (opioids, sedatives, alcohol and others), hypoglycemia, and hypotension.

Weakness of the respiratory muscles

Causes – Causes include neuromuscular diseases like myasthenia gravis, poliomyelitis, botulism, Guillain-Barré syndrome, and drugs affecting the neuromuscular system. Causes of respiratory muscle fatigue include hyperventilation from hypoxemia or metabolic acidosis.

Clinical features – Patients in respiratory arrest are often unconscious or quickly become unconscious. Other features are hypoxemia, which may be associated with cyanosis. Patients with anemia or cyanide or carbon monoxide poisoning do not have cyanosis, even in the face of hypoxemia.

Aspiration

Causes – Causes include swallowing impairments from neurologic and neuropathic diseases, impaired consciousness or cognition, severe vomiting, enteral feeding tubes, endotracheal tubes, oropharyngeal and nasopharyngeal airways, and gastroesophageal reflux disease.

Clinical features – Dyspnea, fever, cough, and chest pain. Features of chemical pneumonitis from aspiration of caustic poisoning include hemoptysis; fever; frothy, pink sputum; wheezing; and diffuse crackles.

Asthma

Causes/risk factors – Causes and/or risk factors include sex; non-Hispanic Blacks; exposure to allergens such as dust, cold, dander, and pollen; diet; and chronic exposure to irritants.

Clinical features – Patients with mild to moderate cases experience chest tightness, breathlessness, wheezing, and cough. Symptoms are often worse during sleep. On presentation, signs include wheezing, tachypnea, pulsus paradoxus, tachycardia, and breathlessness evidenced by the use of accessory muscles of respiration. Patients with severe exacerbations present with altered consciousness, cyanosis, and a silent chest. In chronic cases, patients have barrel-shaped chests and hyperinflated lungs.

Chronic bronchitis

Clinical features – This is characterized by a chronic productive cough that lasts for at least three months over two consecutive years. Smoking is the predominant risk factor for chronic bronchitis. Patients with chronic bronchitis are referred to as blue bloaters and have characteristic cyanosis, edema, chronic productive cough, leg swelling, and pulmonary hypertension.

Emphysema

Clinical features – This is characterized by progressive destruction of the lung parenchyma with loss of elastic recoil, radial airway traction, and alveoli septa. Patients with emphysema are typically referred to as pink puffers. They have a cachectic appearance, pursed-lip breathing, and dome-shaped chest. They also use accessory muscles of respiration.

Smoke inhalation

Causes – These often include acute complications of burns from exposure to fire.

Clinical features – Cough, stridor, and wheezing from local irritation; confusion, coma, and lethargy from hypoxia; and features of carbon monoxide poisoning—headache, weakness, nausea, and confusion.

Chapter 3: Cardiology and Resuscitation

This makes up 20% to 24% of test content. Topic areas include:

Cardiovascular Emergencies

Anatomy of the cardiovascular system

The chambers of the heart

Right atrium

The right atrium receives blood from the superior and inferior vena cava. The superior vena cava drains deoxygenated blood from the head, neck, and upper limbs, while the inferior vena cava drains deoxygenated blood from the abdomen and lower limbs.

Right ventricle

Blood from the right atrium enters the right ventricle and from there is transported into the lungs via the pulmonary artery.

Left atrium

Oxygenated blood enters the left atrium via the pulmonary veins.

Left ventricle

Blood from the left atrium enters the left ventricle, then is transported into the systemic circulation via the aorta.

Valves of the heart

The valves of the heart include two atrioventricular valves, the tricuspid and bicuspid valves, and two semilunar valves (the pulmonic and aortic valves). The heart valves are lined with the endocardium, which is continuous with the chambers of the heart. The heart valves have cusps or flaps that prevent the backflow of blood. The mitral, or bicuspid, valve has two leaflets and is located between the left atrium and left ventricle. It prevents the backflow of blood into the right atrium during diastole.

The tricuspid valve has three leaflets—anterior, septal, and posterior. It is located between the right atrium and right ventricles and prevents backflow of blood during diastole. The pulmonary valve has right, anterior, and left cusps and is located between the right ventricle and the pulmonary trunk. It prevents the backflow of blood into the right ventricle.

The aortic valve is located between the right ventricle and the aorta and prevents the backflow of blood into the right ventricle.

The great vessels of the heart

Superior vena cava

The superior vena cava is a large, short vein that carries deoxygenated blood from the upper limbs, neck, and head. The jugular vein, thyroid veins, and left and right subclavian veins empty into the superior vena cava. The lymphatic duct drains into the subclavian veins. It is responsible for the circulation of lymph in the plasma.

Inferior vena cava (IVC)

This is the largest vein. It drains deoxygenated blood from the lower limbs, abdomen, and pelvis into the heart. It is formed by the confluence of the right and left common iliac veins. The IVC starts posterior to the abdomen in proximity to the aorta in the abdomen. On its way toward the right atrium, the hepatic veins, renal, lumbar, and suprarenal veins drain into it.

Aorta

This is the largest artery. Blood from the left ventricle enters the aorta through the aortic valve. The aorta has a large quantity of elastin that makes it stretch in response to blood volume and pressure. The aorta expands as the ventricle expels blood through the aortic valve. This pressure is necessary to propel blood and maintain pressure in the diastolic phase. This also creates a pressure gradient in which blood in areas of high pressure flows to areas with low pressure.

Parts of the aorta

The arch of the aorta has baroreceptors and chemoreceptors that respond to changes in pressure, pH, and carbon dioxide. Impulses from the chemoreceptors and baroreceptors are transported to the medulla oblongata. The response is then mediated via the sympathetic and parasympathetic nervous systems via the plexus of nerves. From the heart, the aorta travels downward in proximity to the inferior vena cava.

The ascending aorta is between the aortic arch and the heart. It branches into the septic sinuses, then forms the coronary arteries.

The arch of the aorta is the highest part of the aorta. It branches into the left subclavian artery, the left carotid artery, and the brachiocephalic trunk.

The descending aorta is a component of the aortic arch. It branches into the common iliac arteries, which divide further into the abdominal and thoracic branches of the aorta.

The thoracic part, which is a branch of the descending aorta, divides into the esophageal, mediastinal, esophageal, bronchial, and phrenic arteries.

The abdominal aorta, which is a branch of the descending aorta, breaks into the iliac arteries and the renal and suprarenal arteries.

The thoracic aorta is susceptible to aneurysms.

The pulmonary arteries

These arteries transport deoxygenated blood from the right ventricle into the capillaries in the alveoli. These are the only arteries that carry deoxygenated blood. The right and left pulmonary arteries are wide and short, and they deliver blood from the lungs to the heart.

The pulmonary veins

The pulmonary veins are the only veins that carry oxygenated blood. Four pulmonary veins open into the left atrium. Together with the pulmonary arteries, they make up the pulmonary circulation.

Cardiac electrophysiology

The cardiomyocytes can depolarize and repolarize. These actions cause generalized and synchronized contractility of the cardiomyocytes. The heart can generate the initial electrical impulse needed for depolarization. This impulse is generated from the pacemaker cells (the sinoatrial nodes located in the right atrium). The pacemaker initiates a cardiac impulse. This impulse travels to the atria and is transferred to another group of specialized cells called the atrioventricular nodes.

The atrioventricular septum, which is located in the septa between the two atria, conducts impulses from the atria into the ventricles. A delay of about 0.1 second allows the ventricles to contract after the atria have contracted, allowing blood in the atrium to empty into the ventricles. From here, the cardiac impulse is transported to the Bundle of His, a group of specialized cells in the ventricles. The right and left branches of the Bundle of His are located in the interventricular septum. After this, the cardiac impulse is transferred to the apex of the heart via the Purkinje fibers. The impulses are finally shunted to the lateral aspects of the heart.

The arrangement of cells causes the heart to contract synchronously during systole and relax during diastole. A cardiac cycle is characterized by atrial systole and atrial diastole and the ventricular systole and ventricular diastole.

In the cardiac cycle, the opening and closing of the valves are regulated by the rise and fall of the pressure in the heart chamber. However, the pressure in the left side of the heart is higher than that in the right.

Atrial systole

In this phase of the cardiac cycle, there is a filling of the ventricles. A drop in the pressure in the heart causes blood to flow into the atria. When the atria are filled, the atrioventricular valves are opened and about 70% of blood flows into the ventricles. This action is passive. When the atrium contracts, the remaining 30% of blood in the atria is ejected into the ventricles.

Ventricular systole

After atrial systole, the blood in the ventricles is called the end-diastolic volume. In the ventricular systole, the ventricles contract. Increased pressure causes the aortic and pulmonic valves to open. Blood is then ejected into the pulmonary and systemic circulation.

Isovolumetric relaxation

At the end of the ventricular systole, the blood remaining in the ventricles is called the end-systolic volume. The aortic and pulmonic valves close, and pressure in the aorta increases. Meanwhile, the atria go into diastole, fill up with blood, and prepare to commence a new cardiac cycle.

Cardiac output

This is the quantity of blood ejected by the heart in one minute. It is calculated by multiplying the stroke volume (quantity of blood ejected by the ventricles in each heartbeat) by the heart rate. The stroke volume can be calculated by subtracting the ESV from the EDV. Factors that increase stroke volume include exercise, pregnancy, drugs, fever, and more.

Frank-Starling law

This principle states that the preload determines the stroke volume. This preload is the quantity of blood that returns to the heart during ventricular filling. Preload is determined by the amount of blood during ejection. This is also called cardiac output. During ventricular filling, the cardiac muscles stretch. This stretching stimulates cardiac contractility and increases cardiac output. This phenomenon shows a positive relationship between preload and cardiac contractility. However, this phenomenon is limited.

Hormones that increase cardiac contractility include thyroxine and adrenaline. These hormones improve the heart's inotropic function. Calcium channel blockers reduce this function.

Examination of the cardiovascular system

Inspection

On inspection, the patient's appearance is evaluated. The face is inspected for neck pulsations, buccal and conjunctival pallor, and central cyanosis. The fingers are examined for cyanosis, pallor, and finger clubbing, while the lower extremities are examined for pedal edema and clubbing.

Palpation

Pulse

This is caused by contraction of the left ventricle. Increased pressure is felt in the arteries. The pulse can be palpated on the skin surface, where a part of the artery is close to the skin surface or on top of a bone.

Central pulses can be palpated at the carotid artery in the neck and femoral artery in the groin. Peripheral pulses can be felt at the radial artery at the wrist, the dorsalis pedis artery, the brachial artery in the elbow, and the posterior tibial artery.

Blood pressure

Systolic blood pressure is caused by contraction of the left ventricle, while diastolic blood pressure is caused by the relaxation of the ventricles.

Precordium

The anterior chest wall is inspected and palpated for thrills, heart sounds, and murmurs. The parts of the precordium that are examined include the apex at the left ventricle, the pulmonic valve at the upper left part of the parasternum, the aortic valve at the upper right part of the parasternum, and the tricuspid valve at the lower-left area of the parasternum.

When you examine the anterior chest wall, the patient should be supine. A lateral position can change the position of the apex beat. To locate the apex beat, look from the right side of the patient across the fourth to sixth intercostal spaces. Encourage the patient to inhale and exhale slowly. Next, place your right palm on the left precordium, from the fourth to sixth intercostal spaces close to the midclavicular line. If you cannot palpate the apical pulse, move your fingers farther into the anterior axillary line. If you still cannot feel an apical impulse, encourage the patient to roll to the left. If you still cannot feel the impulse, palpate the right side of the anterior chest wall. If the patient has dextrocardia, the apical impulse will be felt.

To palpate the left parasternal region, place the heel of your hand over the left side of the sternum. If there is a pulse or lift present, the duration of the pulse is assessed, along with its character—light or vigorous. To determine the onset, place your right hand over the apex beat and your left hand on the parasternal impulse. A palpable parasternal impulse is a sign of right ventricular hypertrophy. The parasternal impulse is not felt in people with healthy cardiac function.

Palpable murmurs are called thrills. Murmurs from diastolic stenosis and mitral regurgitation can be felt at the apex beat. Aortic stenosis can be felt on the right side of the neck, while pulmonary stenosis is felt on the left side of the neck. The murmurs of a ventricular septal defect are felt in the third and fourth intercostal spaces.

Auscultation

Normal and abnormal heart sounds are heard on auscultation. Auscultation is done after examination of the precordium, carotid pulse, and jugular venous pulse. A stethoscope is used to auscultate the heart.

Components of a stethoscope include the tubing, earpieces, bell, and diaphragm of the chest piece. The bell of the stethoscope is used to hear murmurs with a low frequency, like diastolic murmurs, third heart sound, and fourth heart sound. The diaphragm is used to hear high-pitched sounds, like the first and second heart sounds, aortic regurgitation, and systolic murmurs.

To auscultate

1. Begin from the aortic area. Listen to the first and second heart sounds, aortic regurgitation, aortic stenosis, and aortic ejection.
2. Next, move to the pulmonic area. With the stethoscope diaphragm, assess the aortic and pulmonic sounds, pulmonic stenosis, aortic and pulmonary regurgitation, and pulmonary ejection.
3. At the fourth and fifth intercostal spaces, use the bell of the stethoscope to assess the tricuspid area for tricuspid regurgitation and tricuspid stenosis.
4. Finally, to assess the apex beat, place the diaphragm of the stethoscope at the apex to assess the first and second heart sounds. Also assess for a late systolic click, aortic regurgitation, mitral regurgitation, and an aortic ejection sound.
5. All these should be assessed with the diaphragm of the stethoscope. Place the bell of the stethoscope over the apex beat and put the patient in the left lateral position. Assess for diastolic murmurs.

To assess the systolic or diastolic phase

1. Palpate the carotid pulse as you auscultate.
2. The pulse is felt at systole. The first heart sound describes the beginning of systole. It has M1 and T1 components.

3. The second heart sound signifies the end of systole and the beginning of diastole. It has an aortic and pulmonic component. S1 is the loudest at the apex.
4. Encourage the patient to do about five push-ups to increase the heart rate, then assess for S3 or S4 gallops. These sounds are heard at the apex.

Other areas that are auscultated include the inferior area of the epigastrium and sternum, the lung fields, the liver, abdomen, sacrum, and interscapular area.

How to assess a patient with cardiac symptoms

1. Check pulse. If it is absent, commence chest compressions using the protocol established by the American Heart Association and local bodies.
2. If the pulse is palpable, do a quick primary assessment (airway, breathing, and circulation).
3. Collect a quick history and do a quick secondary assessment.
4. Put the patient in the cardiac position and give supplemental oxygen.
5. Assess the patient's complaint according to the onset of chest pain; factors that aggravate and relieve chest pain; quality of the chest pain (dull, tearing, sharp, stabbing, etc.); radiation; and duration and severity of the pain.
6. Check other vital signs, like blood pressure, pulse rate, and temperature.
7. Assess if the patient is on a prescription of nitroglycerin.
8. If the patient has a prescription for nitroglycerin, give one dose if the blood pressure is greater than 120 mmHg. Repeat the dose in five minutes if the blood pressure is high. Give up to a maximum of three doses.
9. Reevaluate the patient's vital signs and transport immediately to the ER.

Emergency defibrillation

Emergency defibrillation is a component of the chain of survival created by the American Heart Association (AHA). Other aspects of this chain of survival include early access to emergency care, early advanced cardiac life support, early CPR, and integrated care given after cardiac arrest.

Defibrillation must be done quickly on all patients older than one year with sudden witnessed collapse. In such cases, defibrillation is done with an automated external defibrillator. In patients with unwitnessed cardiac arrest, compressions should be done for two minutes or five cycles before defibrillation. A cycle consists of one shock of AED followed by CPR.

In pediatric patients who are one to eight years old, the responder should use a dose attenuator system to give pediatric doses. If this is not possible, the responder can use the standard AED. Manual defibrillators are ideal for pediatric patients who are less than one year old. If a manual defibrillator is not available, use an AED that has an attenuator system. If this is also not available, the standard AED can be used.

Types of automated external defibrillators (AEDs)
Fully automated external defibrillator – This does not require operation by the EMT. The EMT only needs to turn the machine on.
Semi-automated defibrillator – This has a computer voice assistant that analyzes the patient's cardiac rhythm and tells the EMT what to do to manage it.

Factors that cause inappropriate shock delivery
Human error – Use of AEDs for nonshockable rhythms; inefficient CPR; keeping the AED in a charging state for a prolonged period before use, thereby causing the device to automatically discharge; mismatching the defibrillator cables; using a synchronized mode for ventricular fibrillation; poor maintenance of devices; and lack of skilled personnel.

Examples of shockable rhythms
Ventricular tachycardia

1. Attach the AED to unresponsive and pulseless patients to avoid giving inefficient shocks.
2. There should be no human contact when the patient's cardiac rhythm is being analyzed or when the shock is being delivered.
3. Chest compressions should be stopped when the patient's cardiac rhythm is being analyzed.

Advantages of AEDs

- It is easier to use an AED than perform CPR.
- They are safe to use because they require minimal operation and contact.
- They are lightweight and easy to transport.
- Because modern AEDs do not allow the shocking of patients with heartbeats, the risk of error is low.
- AEDs are a vital component of the chain of survival in providing emergency resuscitation.
- Some defibrillators can be handled remotely through the use of adhesive pads. This technology is safe because defibrillation is done without contact with the patient's skin. It also allows for better placement of the electrodes. The adhesive pads have a large surface area, and EMTs are more confident when using this machine to perform defibrillation.

Standard operating procedure

If there is no advanced life support on the scene, patients should be promptly transported to the ER as soon as they have a pulse. As a rule of thumb, one person should use the defibrillator while the other does CPR on the patient. Before use, the battery and function of the defibrillator must be assessed. Also, all contact with the patient must be removed by stating "clear the patient" before the shocks are delivered.

Guidelines on age and weight

Manual defibrillators are suitable for infants. AEDs with a systemic attenuator can be used if these are not available.

Recurrent ventricular fibrillation

1. If ACLS is unavailable and pulse cannot be palpated, stop driving and quickly administer CPR.
2. Attach the defibrillator and analyze the cardiac rhythm.
3. If shockable, shock the patient.
4. Continue resuscitating the patient as indicated.
5. If you are transporting a conscious patient who suddenly becomes unconscious and pulseless, stop driving.
6. Attach the defibrillator and analyze rhythm.
7. If the defibrillator is booting, commence CPR.
8. Shock the patient once as indicated.
9. Continue resuscitating the patient according to AHA guidelines.
10. If there is no pulse, continue CPR and transport the patient.

Witnessed arrest

Commence defibrillation as soon as possible. If this is not available, commence CPR. Do not check the pulse when analyzing cardiac rhythm.

How to coordinate Advanced Life Support (ALS) personnel when using AEDs

1. The protocols are designed according to the EMS system.
2. Use of AEDs on the scene does not require ALS personnel.
3. ALS personnel should be quickly notified of cardiac arrest.
4. The decision to either transport patients or wait for the intervention of ALS personnel should be in line with local protocols.
5. AEDs should be protected from water. They should also not be operated near metal.
6. Machine maintenance should be routinely performed per the operating manual.
7. At the end of each shift, the EMS checklist should be used to evaluate the machine's functionality.

8. Improper care of the device can cause the defibrillator to fail. This can negatively impact the resuscitation and defibrillation of patients. The most common form of device failure is battery failure. Batteries must be properly maintained, and spare batteries must always be available.

Post-resuscitation care

After defibrillation, the patient's pulse rate and other vital signs are reassessed. Patients can have a pulse, or they may have an absent pulse with shock.

Clinical features and causes of common cardiac emergencies

Acute coronary syndromes

STEMI

ST-elevation myocardial infarction is a serious form of a heart attack in which a major coronary vessel is completely blocked and a portion of the heart does not receive a blood supply.

NSTEMI

Non-ST elevated myocardial infarction is a temporal or partial blockage of the coronary artery. It is not as serious as STEMI.

Angina pectoris

This includes Prinzmetal variant, unstable, and stable angina. Complications include arrhythmias, heart failure, aneurysm, myocardial rupture, mural thrombosis, pericarditis, cardiogenic shock, disorders of the papillary muscle, and postmyocardial infarction syndrome.

Aneurysm/dissection

Aortic dissection

This is the passage of blood through a false pocket between the tunica intima and tunica media.

Causes – These include atherosclerosis, malignant hypertension, acquired connective tissue disorders, hereditary connective tissue disorder, iatrogenic causes from aortic catheterization and aortic valve surgery, and trauma.

Clinical features – Tearing pain in the precordial area that spreads to the scapular, severe hypotension, syncope, arterial pulse deficits between the two limbs, and features of impaired perfusion (stroke, paraplegia, renal insufficiency, and myocardial and intestinal infarction). It is often fatal.

Aortic aneurysm

This includes thoracic or abdominal aneurysms.

Causes – These include atherosclerosis, uncontrolled hypertension, family history of aneurysms, white race, male sex, advanced age, and cigarette smoking.

Clinical features – These are often asymptomatic. Clinical features are usually from compression of surrounding structures or rupture. Major complications are embolization, rupture, and DIC.

Cardiopulmonary arrest

This is the arrest of mechanical activity of the heart and consequent reduction of cardiac output. It requires rapid intervention to reduce the risk of death.

Causes – In adults, the causes are mainly primary diseases of the heart, especially coronary artery disease. Other causes in adults are pulmonary embolism, metabolic derangement, hemorrhage of the splanchnic circulation, and trauma. Causes in infants are obstruction of the airway, drowning, sudden infant death syndrome, and smoke inhalation.

CPR in adults

Airway and breathing

Assessment, clearing, and opening of the airway, use of mouth-to-mouth resuscitation in nonhospital settings, ventilating with a BVM, and/or insertion of oropharyngeal or nasopharyngeal airways where appropriate. Endotracheal intubation may be indicated. Note that compression and use of a defibrillator are prioritized over the airway.

Circulation

Chest compressions, interrupted for at least 10 seconds, are done until defibrillation is accomplished. In adults, the compressions are done to a depth of 5 to 6 cm. During compressions, the ER nurse must notice as the chest recoils during the release phase before starting again. Open chest cardiac compressions may be done for patients with penetrating trauma to the chest. In some facilities, mechanical chest compression devices are used to eliminate errors resulting from human fatigue.

Defibrillation

Ventricular fibrillation and pulseless ventricular tachycardia are shockable and therefore amenable to defibrillation. Defibrillation with direct current cardioversion is more effective than antiarrhythmic drugs. In this procedure, defibrillation pads are positioned in between the clavicle and the second intercostal space, just over the fifth intercostal space. About 120 to 200 joules of energy are used, to a maximum of 360 joules.

Drugs

These include adenosine, atropine, calcium chloride, calcium gluconate, dopamine, dobutamine, glucose, epinephrine, naloxone, magnesium sulfate, norepinephrine, procainamide, and others.

Dysrhythmias

Atrial fibrillation

Afib (AF) is a common type of arrhythmia. In this arrhythmia, there are absent waves before the QRS complex. The heart rate is also irregular.

First-degree heart block

This is a sinus rhythm in which the PR interval lasts more than 0.2 second due to prolonged transmission from the atria to the ventricles.

Second-degree AV heart block

This includes Mobitz Type I (Wenckebach) or Mobitz Type II. In Mobitz Type I block, the PR interval lengthens progressively until the QRS complex drops. In Mobitz Type II, there is an intermittent drop in the QRS complex that is not typical of the Type I pattern. Also, in the Mobitz Type II block, there is no rapid progression to a complete heart block.

Third-degree heart block

This is called a complete heart block. There is a discontinuity between the P and QRS waves. The P-P intervals are usually regular, but they are not related to the QRS complexes.

Ventricular tachycardia

Vtach (VT) is a type of arrhythmia in which there are widened QRS complexes, absent P waves, and an abnormal rate that is more than 100 per minute. This rhythm can quickly turn into ventricular fibrillation and death.

Ventricular fibrillation

In Vfib (VF) arrhythmia, there is a chaotic wave pattern that has no pulse. VF may respond to electrical defibrillation.

Paroxysmal ventricular tachycardia
This presents as a narrow QRS complex and, in some cases, wide QRS complex, retrograde P waves may also be seen. There is also rapid and regular tachycardia.

Sick sinus syndrome
There are numerous possible presentations on ECG, including sinus arrest, sinus bradycardia, sinoatrial block, and bradycardia-tachycardia syndrome.

Torsades de Pointes
This presents with a long QT interval and irregular and rapid QRS complexes, which look like they are twisting around the ECG baseline

Premature beats
This is also called premature ventricular contractions. It presents as broad QRS complexes that are more than 1200 ms with associated discordant T wave and ST-segment changes. These beats occur faster than normal for the incoming sinus wave.

Asystole
Another name for this arrhythmia is a flat line. In this case, electrical activity is absent on the cardiac monitor. The rhythm is responsive to defibrillation.

Heart failure
Right ventricular heart failure (RVF)
In this condition, there is an increase in systemic venous pressure due to the backflow of blood from the IVC and SVC. This increase causes movement of fluid from the intravascular space into the tissue space. Affected patients present with pedal and/or sacral edema, distended neck veins, and ascites. Patients also have tender hepatomegaly, which may manifest with hyperbilirubinemia, elevated hepatic enzymes, and prolonged prothrombin time. Patients with chronic RVF have malabsorption syndromes.

Systolic heart failure
This is characterized by decreased cardiac output and increased pulmonary venous pressure. Increased pulmonary venous pressure leads to increased hydrostatic pressure in the capillary bed and consequent pulmonary edema. Patients often present to the ER anxious and restless with cyanosis, breathlessness, and chest pain. Patients must first be placed in the cardiac position and promptly managed with IV Lasix, supplemental oxygen, anticoagulants, and anxiolytics.

Heart failure with reduced ejection fraction

Causes – These include dilated cardiomyopathy, myocardial infarction, and myocarditis. These conditions predominantly affect systolic function.

Clinical features – These are characterized by left ventricular dysfunction with an increase in diastolic volume and reduction in ejection fraction less than or equal to 40%.

Heart failure with preserved ejection fraction

Causes – Heart failure is often caused by conditions that stiffen the ventricles and make them unable to relax. Some causes include valvular disease, hypertrophic cardiomyopathy, constrictive pericarditis, and amyloidosis.

Clinical features – Diastolic heart failure causes an increase in end-diastolic pressure on exertion or at rest. End diastolic volume is often preserved. The ejection fraction is more than 50%.

Pericarditis

Acute pericarditis

Causes – These include autoimmune infections (mostly viral), inflammation, trauma, myocardial infarction (Dressler's syndrome), radiation therapy, uremia, cancer, and drugs (isoniazid, hydralazine, phenytoin, anticoagulants, and procainamide).

Sub-acute pericarditis

Causes – These are the same causes as acute pericarditis but last longer (from days to weeks).

Chronic pericardial effusion

Causes – These include hypothyroidism (myxedema)and metastases from breast and lung carcinomas, sarcoma, lymphoma, melanoma, and leukemia.

Transient constrictive pericarditis

Causes – These may be idiopathic. They may also be caused by infection or inflammation postpericardiotomy.

Fibrosis of the pericardium

Causes – These include sequelae of purulent pericarditis, tuberculosis, MI, carcinoma, or a disorder of the connective tissue. The condition can also be a complication of hemopericardium caused by insertion of pacemakers, cardiac catheterization, insertion of a central venous line, or rupture of a thoracic aortic aneurysm.

Clinical features – These include inflammation (hyperpyrexia, malaise, weakness, and night sweats); pericardial effusion (muffled heart sounds, cardiac dullness, and change in the cardiac silhouette on chest X-ray); pleurisy; chest pain; tachypnea; pericardial friction rub; nonproductive cough; and cardiac tamponade in massive pericardial effusion.

Constrictive pericarditis presents as elevated ventricular and diastolic pressures and congestion of the peripheral venous system (pedal edema, hepatomegaly, and distension of neck veins). A pericardial knock may also be heard.

Peripheral vascular disease

Peripheral arterial disease

Causes – This is caused by atherosclerosis and occlusion of the vessels in the lower limbs.

Clinical features – The condition may be asymptomatic in mild cases, but patients may also present with intermittent claudication. Clinical features are intermittent claudication, which patients describe as an aching, burning, or heavy sensation in their thighs, calves, hips, or buttocks. This pain is worsened by activity and relieved by rest. On examination, the affected limb shows dependent rubor and pale and atrophic hairless skin in chronic cases. The leg may be cyanotic and diaphoretic.

In severe cases, patients present with peripheral arterial ulcers on the heel or toes. The ulcers are tender and have dry, black, and necrotic tissue. Treatment includes removal of risk factors and treatment of underlying cause (smoking cessation, use of antilipids, weight loss, and diet modification); drug therapy with antiplatelet drugs; analgesics; and ACEIs. Surgical intervention includes percutaneous transluminal angioplasty, revascularization, and sympathectomy for amputation in severe cases.

Raynaud's syndrome

Clinical features – This is characterized by vasospasms of arteries in the hands due to cold or emotional stress. Clinical features are paresthesia in the affected hand, characterized by burning, tingling, or cold sensations and pain; change in color; pallor, cyanosis, or rubor.

Secondary Raynaud's syndrome can cause ulcerative changes. Treatment is avoidance of triggers, relaxation techniques, cessation of smoking, and calcium channel blockers. In secondary causes, surgical debridement of the wound may be indicated.

Peripheral venous disorders

Deep vein thrombosis

This is a primary cause of pulmonary embolism. It is characterized by the formation of blood clots in the deep veins of the lower limbs.

Causes/risk factors – These include obesity; patient age greater than 60 years; cigarette smoking; cancers; use of estrogen agonists like tamoxifen; heart failure; hypercoagulability disorders; immobilization; trauma to the limbs; presence of a venous catheter; nephritic syndrome; oral contraceptives or estrogen replacement therapy; prior history of thromboembolism; pregnancy; myeloproliferative neoplasms like polycythemia; sickle cell anemia; and trauma.

Clinical features – Clinical features are asymptomatic in small veins. In bigger veins, they may present as edema, tenderness, and erythema of the affected side. Patients may present with fever or features of pulmonary embolism and thromboembolism.

Arteriovenous fistula

An abnormal communication between an artery and a vein.

Causes – These can be congenital or a result of trauma.

Clinical features – The condition presents as symptoms and signs of arterial or venous insufficiency. Treatment modalities are the use of percutaneous occlusion techniques and surgery.

Varicose veins

The dilation of superficial veins in the lower limbs.

Clinical features – These are often asymptomatic. However, patients may complain of pain, hyperesthesia, and paresthesia in the affected limb. Treatment modalities include compression stockings and surgery.

Composition of the blood

Blood contains plasma, white blood cells, red blood cells, and platelets. These components help blood transport oxygen and nutrients to cells, transport waste and toxins for excretion, form blood clots and control bleeding, fight infection, regulate temperature and hormones, and other mechanisms required for homeostasis.

The composition of blood is 55% plasma (water) and 45% cells. Blood makes up 8% of total body weight. On average, males have about 12 pints of blood, while females have about 9.

Plasma

Plasma is the liquid component that contains water, protein, sugar, fat, and salts. Plasma is a medium for transporting blood cells, hormones, nutrients, clotting factors, antibodies, waste products, and more.

Red blood cells (RBCs)

RBCs, also called erythrocytes, are bright red due to their iron content. They are the most abundant cells in the blood and form about 45% of the blood volume. RBCs are biconcave cells with a flat center. This structure makes them pliable and compressible as they pass through arterioles, venules, and capillaries.

The production of RBCs is controlled by erythropoietin, a hormone secreted by the kidneys that stimulates the release and maturation of blast cells in the bone marrow. Because RBCs have no nuclei, they can change shape as they pass through small blood vessels. However, their annucleation gives them a short half-life of about 120 days.

The function of RBCs is the circulation of oxygen. RBCs contain hemoglobin, which readily binds to oxygen molecules and carbon dioxide. Oxygenated blood, which is carried by the arteries (except the pulmonary artery), is bright red. Deoxygenated blood is dark red. Hematocrit is the percentage of red blood cells in the blood volume. It is used to diagnose anemia.

White blood cells

White blood cells are also called leukocytes. Unlike RBCs, white blood cells make up only 1% of the blood volume. White blood cells protect the body from diseases by fighting bacterial, viral, parasitic, and fungal infections. The most common white blood cells are neutrophils; they make up 70% of the white blood cell count. Because neutrophils are the first to respond to infections, they have a very short life span.

The second most common white blood cells are lymphocytes. T lymphocytes confer cellular immunity and mount a direct attack on antigens, while B cells confer humoral immunity and mount attack via the complement system and antibodies.

Platelets

Platelets, also called thrombocytes, are responsible for hemostasis and control of bleeding. They do this by an interplay of clotting factors, inflammatory mediators, and growth factors.

There are two pathways by which the clotting mechanism is activated: extrinsic and intrinsic. These pathways lead to the activation of thrombin. Thrombin activates fibrin, which in turn polymerizes and forms a platelet plug. A high number of platelets can cause pathologic clotting, while low levels of platelets cause prolonged bleeding.

Thromboembolic diseases

Disseminated intravascular coagulation

This is excessive generation of thrombin in the blood, leading to embolism. When the clotting factors are exhausted, bleeding ensues.

Causes – These include obstetric complications, including abruptio placentae, eclampsia, severe preeclampsia, embolism of amniotic fluid, a retained product of conception, and severe maternal sepsis; septicemia caused by gram-negative microorganisms; adenocarcinomas of the pancreas and prostate; shock; snake envenomation; intravascular hemolysis; tissue damage from burns or frostbite; and complications of prostate surgery.

Myeloproliferative disorders

These include essential thrombocythemia caused by a primary increase of platelets; polycythemia vera caused by a primary increase of red blood cells, white blood cells and/or platelets; primary myelofibrosis; and chronic myeloid leukemia.

Thrombotic disorders

Causes – Genetic causes include protein C deficiency, protein S deficiency, protein Z deficiency, antithrombin deficiency, and mutation of Factor V. Acquired causes are antiphospholipid antibodies; heparin-induced thrombocytopenia; hyperhomocysteinemia; severe sepsis; oral contraceptives; stasis of venous blood; tissue trauma; cancers of the lung, stomach, colon, and pancreas; and atherosclerosis.

Shock

Shock is characterized by hypoperfusion of end organs, dysfunction of the cells, and cell death. Mechanisms involved in shock include decreased cardiac output, hypovolemia, and vasodilation.

Clinical features – These include hypotension, tachycardia, altered consciousness, and oliguria.

Types of shock
Hypovolemic shock
In hypovolemic shock, the intravascular volume is reduced. This reduces preload, which in turn reduces ventricular filling and stroke volume.

Causes – Common causes of hypovolemic shock are hemorrhage from trauma, upper or lower GI bleeding, ruptured aortic aneurysms, and surgeries. Hemorrhage can be concealed, such as a ruptured ectopic pregnancy, or overt, such as hematemesis. Other causes include inadequate fluid intake; dehydration; metabolic acidosis; fever; gastroenteritis; excess use of diuretics; and third space losses such as burns, crush injuries, acute pancreatitis, intestinal obstruction, and myocardial infarction.

Distributive shock
Septic shock causes the redistribution of fluids from intravascular space into tissue spaces.

Causes – The release of toxins into the bloodstream incites an immune response characterized by massive dilation of both arteries and veins. In septic shock, the blood volume is normal. Therefore, resuscitation with IV fluids is not therapeutic. In septic shock, the capillary beds are bypassed. This causes hypoperfusion of end organs and tissues, as well as cellular dysfunction. Apart from sepsis, other causes of distributive shock include anaphylaxis, neurogenic shock, beta-blockers, nitrates, and opioids.

Cardiogenic shock
In cardiogenic shock, cardiac output is reduced due to direct trauma or pathophysiology of the heart. An obstructive shock is a form of cardiogenic shock in which mechanical factors impair ventricular filling and emptying.

Causes – These include aortic regurgitation, dysfunction of prosthetic valves, myocardial infarction, myocarditis, drugs, arrhythmias, and ruptured interventricular septum. Causes of distributive shock include pulmonary embolism, cardiac tamponade, tension pneumothorax, and compression of the vena cava.

Compensated shock
In compensated shock, the body adjusts to cellular hypoperfusion by increasing blood pressure and cardiac output to vital organs. To do this, the heart rate is increased. The respiratory rate is increased, and bronchioles dilate to improve oxygen saturation. Blood flow to the skin is reduced as blood is shunted to the brain, kidneys, and heart.

Clinical features – On examination, there is tachycardia and tachypnea, and the skin is cold and clammy.

Decompensated shock

As tissue perfusion worsens, lactic acid accumulates in the cardiomyocytes and the heart is unable to meet up with oxygen demand. Heart rate, blood pressure, and cardiac output are reduced. Blood floods the tissue spaces.

Clinical features – On examination, there is hypotension, tachycardia, prolonged capillary refill, and thin and thready pulse. The patient is also restless, confused, and agitated.

Irreversible shock

Failure of the compensatory mechanisms causes cell death. Vital organs fail due to the accumulation of carbon dioxide, calcium, and lactic acid. Disseminated intravascular coagulation starts.

Evaluation of the patient in shock

Primary assessment

1. Assess airway patency and position accordingly.
2. Assess respiratory rate and type of respiration.
3. Give supplemental oxygen if necessary.
4. Control external hemorrhage if possible.
5. Assess pulse rate and blood pressure.
6. Assess temperature, hydration status, and skin color.
    - Pale skin shows insufficient tissue perfusion.
    - Cyanosis shows insufficient oxygenation.
    - Cool skin shows vasoconstriction.
    - Mottled skin shows decompensated shock.
7. In pediatric patients, assess capillary refill time.
8. Check the level of consciousness. In shock, patients are agitated, confused, disoriented, and unresponsive.

Secondary assessment

1. Patients with life-threatening conditions should be quickly transported to the ER.
2. Expose the patient from the neck to the abdomen.
3. Reevaluate the vital signs.
4. Obtain a quick history from eyewitnesses.

General management of shock

1. Maintain patency of the airway.
2. Maintain support of the cervical spine.
3. Maintain airflow.
4. Suction as indicated.
5. Give assisted ventilation and supplemental oxygen as indicated.
6. Position the patient appropriately. Patients with cardiogenic shock should be placed in the Fowler's position.
7. Patients with hemorrhagic shock should be placed in the Trendelenburg position or have the foot of the bed elevated to increase venous return.

Chapter 4: Trauma

This makes up 14% to 18% of test content. Topics include:

Trauma

The top cause of death and disability in young adults in the United States is trauma. Trauma is the third most common cause of death of all ages in the United States and the most common cause of hospitalization in the United States, with more than 90% of admitted cases and 23 to 28 million admissions in a year.

In trauma, the body tissues are damaged by forces beyond their threshold. These forces can compress, bend, or pull tissues beyond their inherent threshold. For example, in vehicular accidents, the kinetic force of the vehicle is converted into work required to stop the car, which crushes it. This work is responsible for the damage to the victims of the crash. The force that causes this damage is doubled when the weight of the car is doubled, and it quadruples when the speed of the vehicle doubles. This means that the velocity of the vehicle has more significance than mass on the extent of the trauma.

For trauma to occur, potential energy has to be converted into kinetic energy. For example, a child on a chair or a tree has potential energy. If they fall, this potential energy is converted into kinetic energy. When the child touches the ground, this kinetic energy is converted into work, which is used to stop the child's movement.

Types of trauma

Blunt trauma

This is the top cause of trauma-related death in the United States.
A common cause of blunt trauma is vehicular crashes (MVC). MVCs cause three kinds of collisions:

First-degree collisions – The vehicle crashes against a hard object.

Second-degree collisions – The passenger crashes against the car's interior.

Third-degree collisions – The passengers' internal organs crash against the solid structures in the body.

Nowadays, passengers are cushioned from impact by technologies like restraint systems, airbags, and components that absorb energy. Airbags are usually activated between 140 and 200 mph.

Types of vehicular crashes include:

Frontal collisions – The front end of a vehicle crashes into the front end of another vehicle. These collisions are usually fatal. It is important to assess if the airbag was deployed, if restraints were used, and if there was an intrusion into the victim's compartment.

Rear-end collisions – A vehicle crashes into the rear end of another vehicle. It is important to assess for whiplash injuries and whether restraints and seat belts were used. These collisions are often caused by panic stops, distraction, inattention, and reduced traction of the tires on the road.

Lateral collisions – Also called side-impact collisions, T-bone, or broadside collisions, the side of the vehicle is affected in this form of collision, which occurs commonly in parking lots and intersections. Accidents are usually fatal.

Rollover collisions – These types of crashes are violent, complex, and a reflection of the victim's interaction with the vehicle, road, and other environmental factors. More than 80% of rollover collisions are single-vehicle collisions.

Blast injuries

This is another cause of blunt trauma. The mechanisms involved in a blast injury include:

Primary blast injuries – These injuries are caused by direct pressure on tissues of hollow organs.

Secondary blast injuries – These injuries are caused by collisions with flying objects.

Tertiary blast injuries – These injuries are caused by the collision of the victims against objects after being thrown by the impact of the blast.

Quaternary blast injuries – These are all other injuries caused by the explosion.

Falls
This is another cause of blunt trauma. It is the most common cause of trauma and the second-most common cause of trauma-related deaths. The severity of a fall injury is determined by the type of surface and height of the fall.

Risk factors for falls include:

Age – The most vulnerable age groups for falls are older adults and children. Older adults have the greatest risk of death from falls. This is because aging causes changes in cognition and sensory and physical stamina that increase mortality and morbidity. Falls in childhood are caused by curiosity, development in cognition, and increasing independence. These causes are often escalated by factors like poor parental supervision, poverty, and an unsafe environment.

Sex – Both males and females are at risk of sustaining injuries from falls. However, males are more likely to experience fatal falls than females due to a high prevalence of hazardous occupations and risk-taking behavior in males.

Other risk factors for falls are unsafe work environments; substance abuse; alcoholism; medical conditions like seizure disorders; medications; poor cognition; and vision and socioeconomic factors like overcrowding, poverty, and young maternal age.

Penetrating trauma
This is an open wound caused by the penetration of soft tissues by objects. Penetrating injuries are the second-most common cause of trauma-related death in the United States. The most common forms of penetrating injuries are stab wounds and gunshot injuries. The mechanisms of penetrating trauma include low-velocity injuries caused by knives, ice picks, broken bottles, etc., and medium- and high-velocity injuries from gunshots and bullets. All these injuries cause bleeding and infection of affected tissues.

Assessment of trauma victims

On presentation, it is important to quickly determine the mechanism of injury and the general condition of the patient, then to prioritize resuscitative measures after a quick primary assessment.

Primary assessment – This includes assessment of airway, breathing, circulation, and neurologic status/disability of the patient. Also, the patient must be removed from the offending environment.

Secondary assessment – This is a quick general examination to look for other comorbidities. A focused examination of affected areas is done. This focused examination is done as the patient is transported to the ER.

As a rule of thumb, patients should be managed in the ER or high-dependence units. It is important to quickly determine the mechanism of injuries, as this will help hasten primary and secondary assessments.

Soft tissue injuries

Anatomy of the skin

The skin has three layers—the epidermis, dermis, and hypodermis.

Epidermis – This is the superficial layer of the skin that protects the other layers from friction, heat, and other extreme physical factors. The epidermis is made up of stratified squamous epithelial cells (keratinocytes). The epidermis is not vascularized, and it depends on the dermis and hypodermis for nutrients and water. The epidermis also contains melanocytes, which are pigment-containing cells that protect the skin from UV radiation.

Dermis – The dermis is thicker than the epidermis. It is vascularized and contains blood vessels, hair follicles, nerves, and sweat glands. It is rich in collagen and elastin fibers and is responsible for keeping the skin turgid and firm.

Hypodermis – This is the deepest layer of the skin. It is largely made up of subcutaneous fat, which is stored for insulation, cellular support, and energy consumption.

Physiology of the skin

Protection – The epidermis protects the body from mechanical forces that can be injurious. It also protects the body from dehydration, microorganisms, infection, thermal factors, and UV radiation.

Sensory – The skin helps us connect with our external environment because it is innervated by a rich supply of nerves that receive, transmit, interpret, and act on tactile stimuli.

Thermoregulation – The hypodermal layer of the skin contains subcutaneous fat that insulates the body from cold. Also, this layer acts as an energy reservoir when the food supply is low.

Biochemistry – The skin is involved in many biochemical functions required to maintain homeostasis, such as synthesizing vitamin D required for calcium and phosphorus metabolism.

Closed soft tissue injuries

Contusion

Also called bruises, a contusion occurs when underlying connective tissue and muscles are damaged without discontinuity.

Causes – These include falls, blast injuries, and other forms of blunt trauma. The overlying skin appears blue or purple due to leakage of blood from traumatized capillaries.

Strain

Causes – This form of injury is caused by the overstretching of a muscle or tendon. Strains commonly affect the hamstrings and muscles in the foot and back.

Sprains

Causes – In sprains, the ligament is injured from overstretching or tearing. The most affected areas are the knees, wrists, and ankles. The severity of sprains is graded from grade 1 to grade 3. In grade 1 sprains, some of the fibers in the ligaments are torn. In grade 2, most of the ligament fibers are torn, while in grade 3, the ligament is torn completely.

Hematomas

Causes – In hematomas, blood collects in tissue spaces due to damage to large vessels like arteries and veins. Blood loss can be massive and may cause shock. Hematomas are caused by blunt or penetrating trauma.

Emergency management

1. Take adequate precautions for substance isolation.
2. Conduct a quick primary survey.
3. Maintain airway and breathing.
4. Assess circulation. If the patient is in shock, commence resuscitative measures.
5. Splint any limb with injuries.
6. Transport the patient immediately.
7. Document care that was given and any significant findings.

Open soft tissue injuries
Abrasion
These are scrapes that involve the epidermis and part or all of the dermis.

Causes – Scrapes are caused by shearing forces from blunt trauma. Although they are not as deep as lacerations, they are painful. Treatment includes wound cleaning and prophylactic antibiotics.

Laceration
Causes – In this injury, the epithelial skin is broken by penetrating forces.

Clinical features – Bleeding and hemorrhagic shock are immediate complications. The patient's cardiovascular status must be evaluated, and hemostasis must be promptly commenced. Because these injuries often occur with other injuries, a primary assessment must be done. More serious injuries that involve the bone or neurovascular bundles must be treated first.

Penetration/puncture
Causes – These wounds are caused by objects with sharp ends.

Clinical features – There may be no external bleeding in some cases, but the patient may be bleeding internally. Examples are stab wounds and gunshot injuries.

Avulsion
In this injury, the tissue is torn away from the body.

Clinical features – In most cases, the three layers of the skin are peeled off. In degloving injuries, there is circumferential avulsion of an extremity.

Amputation
Amputation is the separation of a limb from its attachment.

Clinical features – Amputations can be either complete or partial. Immediate requirements for such patients are hemostasis, control of blood pressure, and control of infection.

Emergency care

1. Isolate the patient from the offending environment.
2. Make the airway patent and assess breathing and circulation.
3. Expose the patient to assess the wound.
4. Control bleeding through external compression.
5. Dress the wound to minimize contamination
6. If the patient is in shock, commence shock protocol.
7. For injuries affecting organs, dress the wound with an occlusive dressing. If abdominal organs are eviscerated, dress the organs with a sterile gauze soaked with sterile water. Do not attempt to put the organs back into the body cavity.
8. If the patient is impaled, do not attempt to remove the penetrating object unless the object penetrates the cheek, blocks the airway, or obstructs chest compressions or transportation. Hold the object in place and stabilize with a dressing.
9. For amputations, dress the amputated extremity in sterile gauze. For complete amputations, wrap the amputated extremity in plastic and keep it cool.
10. Assess for injury to the cervical spine.
11. Immobilize the patient.
12. Assess the patient for air embolism.

Injuries to the head, neck, face, and spine

Head injuries

<u>**Open head injuries**</u>

These include penetrating trauma to the scalp and skull, meninges, and brain parenchyma.

Causes – These injuries are usually caused by stab injuries and gunshot injuries. They can also be caused by blunt trauma that fractures the skull with laceration of the overlying scalp.

<u>**Closed head injuries**</u>

Causes – These injuries are caused by blunt trauma to the head or the head being shaken vigorously (such as whiplash), and experiencing acceleration and deceleration of the brain.

Clinical features – The frontal and temporal lobes of the brain are susceptible to diffuse axonal injury from this kind of trauma. Closed head injuries also include intracerebral hemorrhage, subarachnoid hemorrhage, hematomas in the subdural or epidural spaces, and contusions.

Concussion

Clinical features – In a concussion, there is a transient change in the mental status of the affected person. These changes do not last more than six hours. Some of these changes include confusion, memory loss, and loss of consciousness. Concussion does not cause lesions in the brain parenchyma. However, chronic and repeated concussions can cause microtears.

Brain contusions

Causes – Bruises on the brain parenchyma are caused by either open or closed head injuries.

Clinical features – Large contusions can cause verbal edema and consequently increase intracranial pressure. Neurologic symptoms depend on the location of swelling and compression.

Diffuse axonal injury

Causes – This is caused by deceleration rotational and shearing forces that cause widespread discontinuity of axons and myelin sheath. Shaken baby syndrome is one cause of diffuse axonal hemorrhage.

Clinical features – These injuries do not cause gross lesions in the brain parenchyma. They can, however, cause micro-petechial bleeding into the white matter.

Hematomas

Causes – Hematomas are caused by either closed or open injuries to the head. Blood can accumulate in the brain parenchyma, epidural, or subdural space. In subdural hematomas, blood collects between the arachnoid and dura mater. Acute causes include tearing of the cortical veins or bridging veins, head trauma, cerebral contusion, and epidural hematoma.

Chronic cases of subdural hematoma are mostly seen in alcoholics and elderly patients on anticoagulation therapy. Symptoms are gradual and develop over the weeks.

Epidural hematomas are seen in the space between the dura mater and the skull. They are not as common as a subdural hematoma. Large hematomas are caused by damage to the middle meningeal artery from a fracture of the temporal bone. These hematomas are fatal and require prompt intervention.

Intracerebral hematomas occur in the brain parenchyma. They are formed when multiple contusions coalesce. These hematomas can raise the intracranial pressure and cause herniation of the brain stem.

Skull fractures

Causes – Skull fractures are caused by penetrating injuries. There can, however, be closed injuries that cause skull fractures. Patients with simple linear skull fractures with no other neurologic symptoms are at minimal risk for brain injuries. Patients with these symptoms have an increased risk for intracranial hematomas.

Clinical features – Some forms of skull fractures include depressed fractures, which have a high risk of ripping the dura mater and injuring the brain parenchyma; temporal bone fractures, with an increased risk for epidural hematoma; fractures involving the carotid canal that can cause dissection of the carotid artery; and fractures of the occipital and basilar bone that can damage the structures in the middle and inner ear.

Clinical features of specific types of traumatic brain injury

Epidural hematoma – Worsening headaches, decreased consciousness or altered sensorium, hemiparesis and other signs of focal deficits, and dilatation of the pupils with loss of pupillary reflex (herniation). These symptoms develop over several hours.

Subdural hematomas – Immediate unconsciousness.

Intracerebral hematomas and subdural hematomas – Hemiparesis and other focal deficits, progressive loss of consciousness, increased ICP (projectile vomiting, systolic hypertension, widened pulse pressure, bradypnea, bradycardia, and irregular respiration. Features of decerebrate or decorticate posturing are poor prognostic factors. Transtentorial herniation can cause coma, hemiplegia, Cushing triad, and dilated and unreactive pupils.

Basilar skull fracture – CSF otorrhea or rhinorrhea, hemotympanum, bleeding in the external auditory meatus, bleeding in the mastoid area (Battle sign), bleeding in the periorbital area (raccoon eyes), deafness, anosmia, dysfunction of the facial nerve, and fracture of the cranial vault.

Chronic subdural hematoma – Headaches, confusion, drowsiness, seizures, hemiparesis, and other neurologic deficits.

Long-term symptoms – Amnesia, post-concussion syndrome (dizziness, headaches, fatigue, depression, amnesia, anxiety, apathy, hearing loss, and loss of smell), sleep disturbances, change in behavior, seizure disorders, decreased intellectual ability, ataxia, and motor impairment.

In severe cases of traumatic brain injury, affected patients are in a vegetative state in which they lose self-awareness and consciousness. Sleep-wake cycles and autonomic functions are preserved.

Spinal injuries

Anatomy of the spinal cord

The spinal cord begins from the medulla and ends at the L1-L2, which is the upper part of the lumbar vertebrae. It tapers into the conus medullaris, ends in a vertical sheaf, and forms the cauda equina.

The white matter of the spinal cord contains both ascending and descending myelinated tracts. These tracts convey both sensory and motor impulses. The gray matter is located in the central part of the spinal cord and is H-shaped. It is made up of nonmyelinated fibers and cell bodies.

At the anterior horn of the gray matter are lower motor neurons that conduct impulses through the descending corticospinal tracts. The axial parts of these neurons act as efferent fibers. The anterior horns of the gray matter carry sensory fibers from the dorsal root ganglia, as well as neurons that transmit sensory, motor, and reflex impulses from the dorsal nerve roots to the ventral nerve roots from one level of the spinal cord to the other.

The spinothalamic tracts carry pain and temperature impulses in the contralateral side of the spinal cord, while most of the other tracts carry impulses on the ipsilateral side of the spinal cord. There are 31 pairs of nerve roots in the spinal cord.

Spinal cord injury

Over 12,000 people suffer from injuries to the spine annually in the United States.

Causes – Vehicular accidents are the most common cause of spinal cord injuries (48%), followed by falls (16%), accidents (12%), and sports and occupational hazards (10%).

The common risk factors for these injuries are male sex (more than 80% of victims with spinal cord injuries are male) and age. In older patients, degenerative joint diseases and osteoporosis are responsible for slips and falls. Injuries occur from blunt trauma that injures the ligaments, vertebrae, or the spinal cord itself. These forces can bruise or crush the spinal cord. Injuries are also inflicted by penetrating trauma from stab wounds or gunshots. This form of trauma can also injure the vascular bundles and cause hematomas and ischemia.

Clinical features – The pathophysiology behind these injuries includes edema, ischemia, and tissue necrosis. These processes are enhanced by the release of calcium and glutamate from the injured cells and the release of cytokines and free radicals.

Vertebral injury

Injuries to the vertebrae include fractures to the vertebral body, pedicles, lamina or transverse, articular or spinous processes. Injuries also include dislocations of the facets and subluxations of the ligaments, which can also include rupture of the ligament with fractures. If fractures occur in the cervical spine, fractured bones can pierce the vertebral arteries and cause ischemia of the brain stem.

If the vertebral injury is unstable, the bones and ligaments in the vertebrae permit movement that can compress the spinal cord, limit blood flow, and cause severe pain. It can also worsen the patient's neurologic function.

Cauda equina injury

This injury to the lower end of the spinal cord can cause symptoms that mimic conus medullaris syndrome.

Features of spinal cord injury

The usual sign of injury to the spinal cord is a neurologic deficit below the level of the injury. The neurologic function above the lesion is usually intact. Physical signs depend on the level of the injury and whether the injury is complete or partial.

Clinical features – Clinical features of lesions in the upper motor neuron include increased muscle tone, exaggerated deep tendon reflexes, exaggerated plantar responses, clonus, a positive Hoffman reflex, and spastic paralysis. The reverse symptoms are seen in lower motor neuron lesions.

Patients with injury to the vertebrae experience back pain. If these patients have other worse injuries that affect consciousness (such as head injuries), they may not experience pain.

Complete injury to the spinal cord

This manifests as complete flaccid paralysis, autonomic dysfunction below the lesion, and total loss of reflexes and sensation. If the lesion is higher up in the C5 vertebrae, there is respiratory failure. This is worse if the lesion is at C3.

Damage to the cervical cord can cause hypotension and bradycardia (neurogenic shock). Patients experience hypotension and arrhythmias. Flaccid paralysis evolves to spastic paralysis due to absent descending inhibition. If the cord in the lumbosacral section is spared, the autonomic reflexes in this area recover.

Incomplete injury to the spinal cord

Here, there is a loss of motor and sensory function. The deep tendon reflexes are hyperactive. Depending on the type of injury, motor and sensory function may return. However, if there is rapid edema of the spinal cord, there may be a complete loss of spinal function (spinal shock). Features of incomplete injury depend on the part of the cord that is affected. Some examples of spinal cord syndromes include:

Brown-Séquard syndrome

Causes – This is caused by a unilateral transection of the cord.

Clinical features – Patients experience spastic paralysis and loss of proprioception on the same side and loss of temperature and pain sensations on the contralateral side.

Anterior cord syndrome

Causes – This is caused by trauma to the anterior part of the spinal cord or anterior spinal artery.

Clinical features – Patients experience loss of pain and motor sensation on both sides below the injury. However, vibration and proprioception are preserved.

Central cord syndrome

Causes – This is caused by degenerative changes in the cervical spine after injury.
Clinical features – Patients experience impaired motor function in both arms. If there are lesions in the posterior column, patients experience loss of light touch, posture, and vibration. If there are lesions on the spinothalamic tracts, patients lose deep touch, light touch, temperature, and pain sensations.

Accumulation of blood in the cord causes lesions in the lower motor neurons. This manifests as muscle wasting, diminished sensations, and fasciculation. There is also a loss of temperature and pain sensation.

Lesions in the cauda equina

There is a loss of motor and sensory function in the distal limbs.

Clinical features – Sensory loss is asymmetric and is reduced in the perineum (saddle anesthesia). Patients also experience bladder and bowel dysfunction, retention, incontinence, and erectile dysfunction.

Complications of spinal cord injury

Late-onset complications depend on the level and severity of the injury. Respiratory failure occurs in lesions at or higher than C5. Immobility increases the risk of muscle wasting, bone loss, urinary tract infections, pneumonia, atelectasis, pressure ulcers, contractures, and spasticity. Neurogenic shock and dysreflexia occur in injuries to the cervical spine. Chronic paresthesia and neurogenic pain also occur.

Emergency care

1. Take appropriate precautions to isolate infections.
2. Fit the patient with the appropriate cervical collar and reduce movement of the spine.
3. Commence primary survey.
4. Control airway after stabilizing the neck.
5. Assess breathing and circulation (pulse and heart rate).
6. Assess motor and sensory function of all extremities.
7. Do a rapid extrication for severely injured patients.
8. Assess the other parts of the body during the secondary survey.
9. Reassess vital signs and neurologic function.
10. Transport the patient.

How to immobilize the spine

1. All patients with a suspected spinal injury should be immobilized.
2. An appropriately sized cervical collar should be used. An inappropriately sized collar can worsen the spinal injury. The collar should not obstruct the airway.
3. If there is no appropriately sized collar, use a rolled-up towel to support the head.

Indications for rapid extraction

1. The patient is unstable.
2. The scene is unsafe.
3. The patient hinders access to other patients with more severe injuries.

Helmets should be removed during the primary survey. This is done to maintain a patent airway and enable medical professionals to suction patients and perform BVM ventilation.

The helmet may be left in place if it fits the patient's head and does not move, if the removal will worsen the spinal injury, or if the patient's spine can be quickly and directly immobilized with the helmet in place. The helmet must be removed if it restricts the patient's airway, making it difficult to assess the airway; if there is a cardiac arrest; if the patient's spine cannot be properly immobilized with the helmet; and if the helmet does not fit properly.

Children and infants should be immobilized on an appropriately sized board. The shoulders and heels of these age groups should be padded. The appropriately sized cervical collar should be used. If this is unavailable, a rolled-up towel should be used to support the head manually.

Injuries to the eye

Anatomy of the eye

Sclera – This is the outermost layer of the eye. It is avascular and protects the eye.

Choroid – This is the middle layer of the eye. It is highly vascularized and provides nutrients and oxygen to the retina and sclera. It also replenishes the aqueous and vitreous humor.

Retina – This is the innermost layer of the eye. It is highly innervated and is responsible for sending light impulses to the brain via the optic nerve.

Cornea – This is responsible for transmitting and focusing light into the retina.

Lens – This directs light to the retina. Its size is controlled and adjusted by the ciliary body.

Ciliary body – This is a muscle that helps to control the shape of the lens. It is posterior to the iris.

Iris – This is the pigmented part of the eye. It controls the amount of light that reaches the retina.

Pupil – This is located in the center of the iris. Its size is controlled by the oculomotor nerve. It adapts to the intensity of light entering the eye.

Macula – This is located in the retina. It has specialized light-sensitive cells. It degenerates with age.

Fovea – This is the center area of the macula responsible for sharp vision.

Optic nerve – This is a bundle of nerve fibers coming from the retina. It transmits light impulses to the occipital part of the cerebral cortex.

Vitreous humor – This is a gelatinous substance that keeps the eye globular. It fills up the center part of the eye.

Abrasions

Causes – These include contact lenses, foreign bodies lodged in the upper eyelid, and entropion.

Clinical features – These include tearing, redness, foreign body sensation, and discharge from the eyes.

Treatment

1. Use of ophthalmic ointments like bacitracin. Patients who use contact lenses are given antibiotics that cover pseudomonas infections.
2. The pupil is dilated with a cycloplegic to reduce eye pain.
3. Eye patches are not used due to the risk of infections. Also, ophthalmic corticosteroids increase the risk of fungi growth in the eye and reactivation of the herpes simplex virus.
4. Patients are discouraged from wearing contact lenses until the ulcer is completely healed.

Burns

Causes – These include thermal burns from heat and chemical burns from alkalis and acids. Ocular burns from chemicals are usually caused by occupational hazards, assaults, and abuse. Ocular burns from acids are less extensive than burns from alkalis because the acids denature and coagulate the proteins in the eye, thereby preventing further absorption of the acids. Alkalis, on the other hand, liquefy the eye proteins and penetrate underlying tissues, thereby causing more extensive burns.

Treatment – Thermal burns involve more of the eyelids because of the blink reflex. The eyelids are irrigated with copious amounts of normal saline, then dressed with antimicrobial ointment. Thermal burns to the eye are usually mild. Patients are managed with antimicrobial ointment, cycloplegics, and oral analgesia.

In chemical burns, the eyeballs and eyelids are irrigated with copious amounts of normal saline or a borate buffer solution under local anesthesia. Irrigation is done until the pH of the cornea is normal.

Burns are managed with ocular antibiotics and cycloplegics. Ocular corticosteroids are used only at an ophthalmologist's discretion. An ophthalmologist should be promptly consulted to reduce the risk of perforation, globe rupture, scarring, and deformities of the eyelids.

Foreign bodies

Causes and clinical features are the same for corneal abrasions as discussed above.

Treatment – Surface foreign bodies are managed with irrigation or manual removal under ocular anesthesia by an ophthalmologist. Intraocular foreign bodies are removed surgically by an ophthalmologist. Thereafter, ocular and systemic antibiotics are used. Ointments are not used if there is a rupture of the globe.

Retinal detachment

Causes/risk factors – Risk factors for rhegmatogenous detachment are myopia, ocular trauma, cataract surgery, family history of retinal detachment, and lattice retinal detachment. Risk factors for traction retinal detachment are sickle cell retinopathy and diabetic retinopathy. Risk factors for serous detachment are cancers, choroid, choroidal hemangiomas, and severe uveitis.

Clinical features – Retinal detachment is often painless. In the early stage, patients experience vitreous floaters, blurred vision, and photopsia. In the late stages, patients experience grayness in the visual field. If the macula is involved, the central vision is affected. In the ER, patients present with retinal hemorrhage as a result of trauma.

Treatment – Treatment options are vitrectomy, scleral buckling, sealing of the retinal breaks, and pneumatic retinopexy.

Trauma

Hyphema – This is bleeding in the anterior chamber from blunt trauma to the eye. Immediate complications are raised intraocular pressure, glaucoma, recurrent bleeding, and permanent blindness in the affected eye.

Immediate measures include placing the patient in the semi-Fowler's or high Fowler's position and the use of an eye shield to protect the eye. Intraocular pressure is monitored and controlled with the appropriate drugs (brimonidine and timolol). Corticosteroids are administered to reduce inflammation. Aminocaproic acid or tranexamic acid may be used to control recurrent bleeding.

Globe rupture – Immediate interventions for laceration of the globe include using an eye shield to protect the eyes, reduction of intraocular pressure, and systemic antibiotics to treat infections. Topical antibiotics are avoided. Because vomiting can increase IOP, antiemetics are used. Corticosteroids are not used until the wounds are closed surgically. Tetanus prophylaxis is also given. An ophthalmologist must be consulted immediately.

Anatomy of the face

There are 14 bones in the face. The only movable bone is the mandible. Because the face is highly vascularized, minor traumas can cause bleeding. Apart from hemorrhage, trauma to the face can obstruct the airway.

Injuries to the face

Causes – These injuries are usually caused by vehicular accidents (75%). Life-threatening scenarios occur when the airway is obstructed. Cervical injuries can occur with facial trauma.

Emergency care

1. Stabilize the cervical spine.
2. Inspect the oral cavity and remove foreign bodies, broken teeth, and avulsed tissue.
3. Suction if necessary.
4. Give supplemental oxygen via PPV or an NRB.
5. Use external compression for hemostasis.
6. Package any avulsed tooth in gauze soaked with saline.
7. Treat for shock if appropriate and transport.

Injuries to the nose

1. Use compression for external bleeding.
2. For epistaxis, seat the patient and encourage the person to pinch their nose.
3. Nasal fractures should be treated with cold compression.

Injuries to the ear

1. Use compression for external hemorrhage.
2. Wrap any avulsed tissue with saline-soaked gauze.
3. Do not pack the ear.

Injuries to the neck

1. Immobilize the patient and do a primary survey and assessment.
2. Cover the neck injuries with an occlusive dressing.
3. Quickly transport the patient to an ER unit.
4. For injured blood vessels, cover with an inclusive dressing and apply light pressure for compression.
5. Secure the dressing with gauze strapped around the shoulder and axilla.
6. Quickly transport the patient lying on the left side. The head should be tilted down.
7. Give oxygen and monitor for shock.

Trauma to the chest

Anatomy of the chest

The chest is made up of the thoracic spine, ribs, muscles, fat, neurovascular bundles, and skin. It protects the heart, lungs, and liver, and it supports the upper extremities and shoulder. Even if the thoracic spine is bony, its connection to muscles makes it flexible enough to permit expansion of the chest wall during inspiration.

The surface landmarks of the anterior chest wall include the sternal notch and nipple. The mid sternal line is measured from the sternal notch to the xiphoid process. The landmark of the lateral sternal line is down the lateral border of the sternum. It is used in locating the internal thoracic artery. The midclavicular line is identified from the middle part of the clavicle down to the medial side of the nipple. This landmark is used in performing a thoracostomy.

The superior boundaries of the axilla include the outer part of the first rib, the superior part of the scapula, and the middle third part of the clavicle. The lower border of the axilla makes up the inferior boundary. The anterior border is made up of the pectoralis major and minor, while the posterior border is made up of the latissimus dorsi.

The anterior axillary line, which is used in placing a chest tube, is drawn from the anterior axillary border down to the chest wall. The posterior axillary line is drawn down from the posterior axillary border to the chest. The midaxillary line is drawn from the apex of the axilla.

The skeleton of the thorax is made up of 12 thoracic vertebrae (T1-T12/posterior aspect), 12 pairs of ribs (lateral and anterior), and a sternum (medial and anterior).
The first seven ribs are called true ribs because they attach to the manubrium and sternum. The eighth, ninth, and tenth ribs are called false ribs because their costal

cartilages join to connect to the sternum through the costal arch. The eleventh and twelfth ribs are called floating ribs.

The sternum is made of three bones: the manubrium, the sternal body, and the xiphoid process. The sternum acts as a pivot for the attachment of muscles.

The muscles of the chest wall include the intercostal muscles, which move the ribs; the transversus thoracis; the pectoralis major and minor; and the serratus anterior.

The neurovascular structures are located in the inferior border of each rib in the costal groove. During thoracentesis and thoracostomy, the costal space is entered via the superior border. The ribs are nourished by the intercostal branches of the internal thoracic artery (a branch of the subclavian artery). The anterior chest wall is innervated by the medial and lateral pectoral nerves (branches of the brachial plexus).

Trauma

About 25% of trauma-related deaths in the United States are caused by thoracic trauma. Most chest injuries are fatal, and death can occur in minutes. Chest injuries can be from either penetrating or blunt forces. Fractures to the ribs and clavicle are very common compared to fractures of the scapula and sternum. There can also be associated injuries to the diaphragm and esophagus. Injuries below the nipple can affect abdominal structures.

Pathophysiology of chest trauma includes respiration and circulation. Respiration is affected by trauma to the lungs or airway (tracheobronchial disruption and constriction of the lungs) and ineffective respiration patterns (pneumothorax, hemothorax, and flail chest).

Circulation is affected by hemorrhage and shock, decreased venous return and cardiac output, and direct injury to the heart. Increased thoracic pressure reduces venous return (tension pneumothorax, massive hemothorax, and cardiac tamponade). Blunt injuries to the lungs can cause heart failure and arrhythmias. Late-onset complications include pneumonia and atelectasis.

Flail chest

Causes – These include fractures of more than three adjacent ribs from blunt or penetrating trauma. The broken ribs move paradoxically during breathing (inward during inspiration and outward during expiration).

Treatment – This includes acute resuscitation and stabilization for patients with multiple injuries.

Hemothorax

Causes – These include accumulation of blood within the pleural space due to penetrating injuries that lacerate the lung, internal mammary artery, or intercostal vessels.

Clinical features – In large hemothoraces, patients present with difficulty breathing. On examination, there are decreased percussion notes and breath sounds on the affected side. These may not be easily elicited in patients with multiple injuries. Patients may also present with hypovolemic shock.

Pneumothorax

Causes – These include penetrating or blunt trauma to the chest. Patients may also present with hemithorax.

Clinical features of traumatic pneumothorax – These include difficulty breathing, tachypnea, pleuritic chest pain, and tachycardia. On examination, there are hyperresonant sounds on percussion and crackles when the affected side is palpated (subcutaneous emphysema). There may also be a Hamman sign caused by air in the mediastinum.

Clinical features of tension pneumothorax – Patients may present with hypotension, distension of the neck veins, and tracheal deviation. The affected area is also tense and distended.

Treatment – This includes acute resuscitation with IV fluids, supplemental oxygen, and mechanical ventilation as indicated. Immediate thoracentesis and chest tube thoracostomy.

Pulmonary contusion

Causes – Blunt or penetrating chest trauma.

Clinical features – These include chest pain, difficulty breathing, and tenderness of the chest wall. Complications are acute respiratory distress syndrome and pneumonia.

Treatment – Acute resuscitation with mechanical ventilation where indicated. Supportive management with analgesics and supplemental oxygen.

Aortic disruption

Causes – Rupture of the aorta following blunt or penetrating chest injury.

Clinical features – These include pulse deficits of the upper extremities, chest pain, systolic murmur, hoarseness, hypotension, and shock.

Treatment – This includes acute resuscitation with fluids and supplemental oxygen, and stabilization of blood pressure with a beta-blocker. Definitive treatment is emergency repair or insertion of an endovascular stent.

Myocardial contusion

Causes – Blunt cardiac injury.

Clinical features – Patients may present with arrhythmias in severe cases.

Rupture of the ventricles

Causes – It is typically caused by a blunt cardiac injury.

Clinical features –Fatal, although patients with smaller tears may present with cardiac tamponade.

Disruption of valves

Causes – It is typically caused by blunt trauma to the chest.

Clinical features – Patients often present with murmurs and features of heart failure.

Septal rupture

Causes – It is typically caused by blunt trauma to the chest.

Clinical features – Patients may present with heart failure.

Commotio cordis

Causes – Typically this is caused by a blunt cardiac injury, such as blunt trauma to the precordium in patients without underlying cardiovascular comorbidity.

Clinical features – Patients present with sudden cardiac arrest. It causes ventricular fibrillation and is often fatal.

Emergency care

Primary survey:

1. Airway – Assess airway for obstruction with foreign bodies, vomitus, or blood. Assess the efficiency of breathing, pulse rate, respiratory rate, and shock.
2. Keep the airway patent.
3. Secure the cervical spine.
4. Suction the airway if necessary.
5. Use an airway device if necessary to keep the airway patent.
6. Provide supplemental oxygen.
7. Assess breathing.
8. Cover injuries to soft tissues with an occlusive dressing.
9. Immobilize the patient and manage for shock.
10. Transport quickly to the ER.
11. For flail segments, stabilize the ribs with your hand first, then use a towel or dressing to splint the chest wall.

Trauma to the abdomen

Anatomy of the abdomen

The abdomen protects the gut, kidneys, and reproductive organs. It is made up of the lumbar spine and muscles that connect the chest to the pelvis.

The lumbar spine has five vertebrae: L1–L5. It makes up the posterior section of the abdomen. These vertebrae are the largest bones in the spinal column and bear weight from the cervical and thoracic spine.

The muscles of the anterior and lateral abdominal wall include the internal and external oblique muscles, transversus abdominis, rectus abdominis, and pyramidalis. These muscles act like a girdle that supports the pelvis and lumbar vertebrae and protects the abdominal organs. The muscles of the posterior abdominal wall include the iliacus, quadratus lumborum, diaphragm, and psoas minor and major. These muscles work with the anterior abdominal muscles to support the lower spine.

The arteries supplying the anterior and lateral abdominal wall are the superior and inferior epigastric arteries, subclavian artery, musculophrenic artery, posterior intercostal artery, superficial epigastric artery, and superficial circumflex iliac artery.

The nerves supplying the anterolateral abdominal wall are the iliohypogastric nerve, ilioinguinal nerve, thoracoabdominal, subcostal, and lateral cutaneous nerves.

Abdominal injuries

Abdominal injuries can be from either blunt or penetrating trauma.

Causes of blunt trauma – A direct impact (assault) or impact from falls or sudden deceleration.

Clinical features – The most commonly affected organs are the spleen, liver, and small intestine.

Causes of penetrating trauma – These include stab injuries or gunshots.

Clinical features – These injuries can reach the peritoneum. Penetrations below the diaphragm can affect intrabdominal organs, like the stomach and liver. There can be associated injuries to the pelvis, spine, ribs, and major vessels, like the inferior vena cava and thoracic aorta.

Lacerations to the abdomen hemorrhage quickly. Hemorrhages from low-grade solid organs or hollow viscus, like the intestine, are often low volume. Heavy bleeding from highly vascularized organs, like the spleen, can cause acidosis, shock, and coagulopathy. This form of hemorrhage is internal (retroperitoneal or intraperitoneal). Lacerations to the viscus—like the intestine, bladder, and stomach—quickly cause sepsis.

Late-term complications include rupture of hematomas, bowel obstruction, biliary leakage, and abdominal compartment syndrome.

Other clinical features of abdominal trauma – These include pain, hemorrhage, hemorrhagic shock, or hypovolemia.

Abdominal evisceration

Trauma to the abdomen causes protrusion of the abdominal viscus.

Emergency care

1. Organs must not be touched with bare hands to prevent contamination.
2. Remove all clothing covering the viscus.
3. Cover the organs with a saline-soaked dressing.
4. Do not try to pack the organs back into the cavity.
5. Cover the dressing with a plastic wrapper.
6. Secure the dressing with tape.
7. Transport promptly to the ER.

Bladder trauma

Causes – These include blunt or penetrating trauma to the pelvis, perineum, or suprapubic region of the abdomen. Blunt trauma is the most common cause following a vehicle crash, an external blow to the abdomen, or a fall. Patients are also likely to have pelvic fractures. The bladder can also be injured during pelvic surgeries—especially abdominal hysterectomy, excision of a pelvic mass, and caesarean section. Risks increase when there is fibrosis from surgery or radiation exposure and when the tumor to be excised is extensive.

Clinical features – These include suprapubic pain, urine retention, and hematuria. Patients may also present with abdominal distension, peritonitis, and hypovolemic shock. Complications are urine ascites, persistent hematuria, infections and sepsis, incontinence, and formation of a fistula.

Genital trauma

Trauma to the male genitalia includes injury to the scrotum, penis, and testes.

Causes – Testicular injuries are sustained from blunt trauma from sports, vehicular accidents, and assault. Penetrating trauma to the testes is not common. Scrotal trauma includes burns, penetrating injuries, and scrotal avulsion. Injuries to the penis can be sustained from sexual activity or assault; entrapment; strangulation; and penetrating trauma from human bites, animal bites, and gunshot injuries. The most common complication is bleeding followed by infection. Other complications are erectile dysfunction, urethral scarring, and hypogonadism.

Trauma to the female genitals includes sexual assault, blunt trauma, traumatic childbirth, insertion of a foreign body, and blunt trauma. These injuries can manifest as avulsions, amputation, crush injuries, hematomas, contusions, and lacerations.

Assessment and care

1. Use external compression to control bleeding.
2. Do not pack a bleeding vagina.
3. Avulsed or amputated tissue should be covered in saline-soaked gauze and transported along with the patient.
4. Use a cold compress to treat pain and swelling.

Orthopedic trauma

Fractures can be either open or closed. In open fractures, the skin is broken and the fracture is exposed. In closed fractures, the skin integrity is preserved.

Causes – Pathologic fractures are caused by mild forces that affect weak or diseased bone tissue (cancer, infection, osteoporosis and bone cyst). Stress fractures are caused by repeated forces on bone (as with long-distance runners). In this case, there is not sufficient time given for bone cells to heal and recover from the repetitive impact.

Complications – Risks for complications increase with open fractures. These kinds of fractures have a higher risk for bleeding, infection, and damage to nerves and blood vessels.

Acute complications of fractures include:

Hemorrhage – Patients with severe hemorrhage experience hypovolemic shock. The risk for this is increased in fractures of the femur and pelvis.

Trauma to blood vessels – Open fractures can damage blood vessels. Some closed fractures, such as fractures of the supracondylar part of the humerus, can also damage blood cells and cause ischemia. In closed fractures, this may not be noticed on time.

Injury to nerves – Nerves can be damaged by direct disruption, compression, or stretching. Temporary nerve damage (neuropraxia) can cause temporary loss of motor and sensory function for about seven weeks. Recovery of damaged nerves can take weeks to years, depending on the type and extent of injuries.

Pulmonary embolism – This fatal complication is high in patients with fractures of the hip or pelvis.

Fat embolism – Fractures of the femur, humerus, and other long bones can cause embolism of fat cells to the lungs.

Compartment syndrome – Crush injuries and comminuted fractures can trigger an increase in tissue pressure. If this occurs in closed circumferential fascia spaces, compartment syndrome occurs. If untreated, tissue necrosis and gangrene rapidly develop.

Infection – This complication is higher in open fractures. Late-onset complications include bone and joint instability, impaired range of movement, bone stiffness, a delayed union of fracture, malunion, osteoarthritis, osteonecrosis, and limb length discrepancy.

Emergency care

1. Do a primary survey.
2. Isolate the body substance.
3. Administer supplemental oxygen if necessary.
4. Assess for other life-threatening injuries. After this, splint the fracture and prepare the patient for transport.
5. If it is an extremity that was fractured, elevate the limb to reduce swelling.
6. Splinting reduces swelling. It also reduces the risk of movement of bone fragments, angulated joints, and bone ends and minimizes the risk of embolism and trauma to blood vessels, muscles, and nerves. It controls bleeding and reduces the risk of paralysis, compartment syndrome, pain, and bone deformity.

How to splint

1. Assess pulse, sensory, and motor function of the distal part of the fracture before and after application of the splint. Document your results.
2. Immobilize the joint below and above the injury.
3. Cover open fractures with sterile gauze.
4. Do not attempt to pack and replace a broken extruding bone.
5. Pad the splints to provide comfort to the patient.
6. Splint patients before transport.
7. Patients with hypovolemic shock should be splinted in the normal position and quickly transported.

Complications of splinting

1. Nerve compression
2. Tissue ischemia
3. Compartment syndrome
4. Worsening pain

How to splint a joint

1. Isolate body substance.
2. Manually stabilize the joint.
3. Assess motor and sensory function and pulse.
4. If the distal part of the fracture is cyanosed or pulseless, align the fracture and apply gentle traction. Immobilize the joint and reassess pulse, motor, and sensory function. Record results of finding.

When to use a traction splint

1. Injury to the knee or close to the knee
2. Injury to the pelvis or hip
3. Fracture with avulsion or partial amputation

How to splint lower leg or ankle injury

1. Assess motor and sensory function and pulse.
2. Isolate the body substance.
3. Manually stabilize the leg.
4. Put the splint under the lower leg and measure the splint to suit the proper length of the lower leg.
5. Secure the straps.
6. Reassess pulse, motor, and sensory function.
7. Immobilize the hip and secure the joint to the board.

Chapter 5: Medical Emergencies

This makes up 27% to 31% of test content. Topic areas include:

Respiratory Emergencies

Aspiration

Causes – These include swallowing impairment from neurologic and neuropathic diseases, impaired consciousness or cognition, severe vomiting, enteral feeding tubes, endotracheal tubes, oropharyngeal and nasopharyngeal airways, and gastroesophageal reflux disease.

Clinical features – These include dyspnea, fever, cough, and chest pain. Features of chemical pneumonitis from aspiration of caustic poisoning include hemoptysis; fever; pink, frothy sputum; wheezing; and diffuse crackles.

Treatment – Supportive treatment includes supplemental oxygen and assisted ventilation. Antibiotic therapy with beta-lactamase inhibitors or clindamycin for patients with chemical pneumonitis. Abscesses in the lungs are treated with IV antibiotics and percutaneous drainage.

Asthma

Causes/risk factors – These include male sex; non-Hispanic Blacks; exposure to allergens such as dust, cold, dander, and pollen; diet; and chronic exposure to irritants.

Clinical features – Patients with mild to moderate cases experience chest tightness, breathlessness, wheezing, and cough. Symptoms are often worse during sleep. On presentation, signs include wheezing, tachypnea, pulsus paradoxus, tachycardia, and breathlessness evidenced by the use of accessory muscles of respiration. Patients with severe exacerbations present with altered consciousness, cyanosis, and a silent chest. In chronic cases, patients have barrel-shaped chests and hyperinflated lungs.

Treatment – Acute resuscitation with supplemental oxygen and NIPPV for patients with cyanosis and metabolic acidosis. Inhaled bronchodilators with beta-agonists, like salbutamol and albuterol, and acetylcholine receptor antagonists, like ipratropium bromide. Nebulized bronchodilators are used for children. IV corticosteroids to reduce inflammation and mucus plug formation in the respiratory tract. Magnesium sulfate for bronchodilation.

Chronic obstructive pulmonary disease

Chronic bronchitis – This is characterized by a chronic productive cough that lasts for at least three months in two consecutive years. Smoking is the predominant risk factor for chronic bronchitis. Patients with chronic bronchitis are referred to as blue bloaters with characteristic cyanosis, edema, chronic productive cough, leg swelling, and pulmonary hypertension.

Emphysema – This is characterized by progressive destruction of the lung parenchyma with loss of elastic recoil, radial airway traction, and alveoli septa. Patients with emphysema are typically referred to as pink puffers with cachectic appearance, pursed-lip breathing, dome-shaped chest, and use of accessory muscles of respiration.

Infections

Community-acquired pneumonia – This pneumonia is transmitted outside the hospital. The most common causative pathogens are Streptococcus pneumonia, Hemophilus influenza and atypical bacteria-like Legionella species, Chlamydia pneumonia, viruses, and Mycoplasma pneumonia.

Nosocomial pneumonia – This is hospital-acquired pneumonia. Risk factors include immunosuppression, intubation, old age, immobility, and sepsis. Nosocomial pneumonia is contracted by inpatients 48 to 72 hours after being admitted. It is generally caused by a bacterial infection rather than a virus. Implicated bacteria include rod-shaped gram-negative organisms like Pseudomonas aeruginosa, Klebsiella pneumoniae, and Enterobacter spp; gram-positive bacteria, like Staphylococcus aureus; and Hemophilus influenzae. Implicated viruses include influenza and respiratory syncytial virus and cytomegalovirus.

Tuberculosis – Risk factors for pulmonary tuberculosis include immunosuppression as seen in cancer, chemotherapy, and HIV. Tuberculosis is caused by Mycobacterium spp.

Empyema – This is the collection of pus/abscesses in the lungs. Risk factors include pulmonary tuberculosis and other infectious suppurative lung diseases.

Ventilator-associated event – This is a new or progressive and persistent radiographic abnormality that develops in a patient on mechanical ventilation or within 48 hours of mechanical ventilation. The patient must also demonstrate one or more systemic signs like fever, leukopenia or leukocytosis, or have altered mental status in patients more than 70 years of age, and have the following pulmonary criteria: dyspnea, rales, new-onset cough, increased respiratory secretions, impaired oxygenation, and bronchial breath sounds.

Inhalation injuries

Irritant gas inhalation injury

Causes – These gases dissolve in water in the respiratory tract and cause inflammation. They include sulfur dioxide, hydrogen sulfide, ozone, ammonia, chlorine, nitrogen dioxide, phosgene, and chloramine, which is obtained by mixing toilet cleaners with bleach.

Acute exposure to these gases in large doses is most often from industrial accidents. Water-soluble gases, like hydrogen chloride and sulfur dioxide, quickly dissolve in the upper airway and stimulate an acute inflammatory response, while less soluble gases, like ozone and phosgene, do not stimulate an acute response until they are properly dissolved in the respiratory tract. They cause a delayed inflammatory response.

Clinical features – Immediate response includes coughing, retching, hemoptysis, wheezing, and chest pain. Irritant gases also irritate the eyes and nose. About two weeks after exposure, some patients experience bronchiolitis obliterans caused by plugging of the airways with granulating tissue. This can lead to acute respiratory distress syndrome. Complications are acute respiratory distress syndrome, superseding bacterial infection, sepsis, and pulmonary fibrosis.

Treatment

1. Removal from exposure and decontamination.
2. Supportive management of symptoms, including supplemental oxygen, inhaled bronchodilators and systemic corticosteroids.
3. In severe cases, patients are managed with mechanical ventilation and inhaled epinephrine.

Smoke inhalation

Causes – Often an acute complication of burns from exposure to fire.

Clinical features – These include coughing, stridor, and wheezing from local irritation; confusion; coma and lethargy from hypoxia; and features of carbon monoxide poisoning—headache, weakness, nausea, and confusion.

Treatment – Supportive with supplemental oxygen and mechanical ventilation. Hyperventilation or use of hyperbaric oxygen is required for carbon monoxide poisoning.

Obstruction

Obstruction of the airway can be due to narrowing and remodeling (asthma and COPD), and alpha-1-antitrypsin deficiency. Other causes of obstruction include tumors of the respiratory tract, pneumothorax, hemothorax, abscess, and others.

Pleural effusion

This is an accumulation of fluid within the pleural space.

Causes – These are varied and classified as either transudates or exudates.

Clinical features – Diagnosis is clinical and confirmed by chest X-ray. However, thoracocentesis and analysis of the pleural fluid are needed to diagnose the cause. Treatment modalities include thoracocentesis, pleurectomy, and chest tube drainage.

Pneumothorax

This is the accumulation of air in the pleural space. Types include primary pneumothorax, which occurs in young men with a tall and thin habitus. There is typically no underlying lung disease. Secondary spontaneous pneumothorax occurs in patients with underlying pulmonary pathology. Traumatic pneumothorax occurs as a result of blunt or penetrating trauma to the chest wall. Iatrogenic pneumothorax occurs as a result of surgical interventions, like thoracocentesis, transthoracic needle aspiration, mechanical ventilation, and others.

Pulmonary edema

Causes – Cardiogenic causes include left ventricular heart failure from decompensated heart failure, acute coronary syndrome, arrhythmia, or valvular disease. Noncardiogenic causes include fluid overload, drowning, aspiration pneumonitis, respiratory distress syndrome, allergic reactions, and acute kidney injury.

Clinical features – These include chest tightness, difficult breathing, chest pain, worsening cyanosis, diaphoresis, and anxiousness. Patients with cardiogenic causes present with cardiovascular symptoms like murmurs, distended neck veins, hypertension, and hepatomegaly.

Treatment

1. Place the patient in the high Fowler's position for relief of chest symptoms. This position causes gravitational movement of fluid to the lower lobes of the lung.
2. Administer supplemental oxygen. Unresolved cases will require mechanical ventilation.
3. Give IV Lasix for cardiogenic causes of pulmonary edema.
4. Give IV morphine to reduce the work of breathing.
5. Give IV inotropes for patients with heart failure.
6. In noncardiogenic causes, the underlying causes are treated.

Pulmonary embolism

Causes/risk factors – Deep vein thrombosis is the most common cause of pulmonary embolism. An embolus is most often released from the deep veins of the legs. However, embolus can come from the central veins of the chest via central lines and thoracic outlet syndromes and the veins in the arm. Risk factors for deep vein thrombosis are discussed in peripheral venous disorders under cardiovascular emergencies.

Clinical features – These include chest pain, difficulty breathing, cough, hemoptysis, and symptoms of shock in massive embolism—hypotension, tachypnea, tachycardia, and features of right ventricular heart failure. Patients may also present with localized features of deep vein thrombosis.

Treatment

1. Acute resuscitation with supplemental oxygen and mechanical ventilation where indicated
2. Rapid dissolution of clots with systemic thrombolytic drugs or catheter-directed therapy
3. Anticoagulation therapy
4. Prevention of further embolism by controlling and modifying risk factors

Respiratory distress syndrome

Causes – These include increased hydrostatic pressure in the alveolar capillaries (pulmonary edema); increased permeability of the alveolar capillaries; diffuse alveolar hemorrhage; right to left cardiac shunts as seen in congenital cyanotic heart diseases; and Eisenmenger syndrome.

Clinical features – These include difficulty breathing, anxiety, restlessness, cyanosis, altered sensorium, diaphoresis, tachycardia, tachypnea, crackles, distended neck veins, cardiac arrhythmia, and death.

Treatment – Mechanical ventilation. Treatment of the underlying cause.

Neurologic Emergencies

Seizure disorders

Causes

Patients less than two years old – Fever, birth injuries, hereditary neurological disorders, and congenital or acquired metabolic disorders
Ages 2 to 14: Idiopathic
Adults: Alcohol withdrawal, trauma, strokes, idiopathic causes
Older people: Strokes and tumors

Classification

Generalized-onset seizures – These include motor and nonmotor (absence seizures). In this disorder, the seizure begins from neurons in both cerebral hemispheres. Patients lose both consciousness and awareness. Patients with generalized motor seizures have bilateral motor activity and are classified into tonic-clonic, clonic, tonic, myoclonic-atonic, infantile spasms, myoclonic, atonic, and myoclonic-tonic-clonic seizures. Generalized nonmotor seizures include typical absence seizures, atypical absence seizures, eyelid myoclonia, and myoclonic seizures. Absence seizures occur in children.

Focal onset seizures – These seizures stake in one cerebral hemisphere or subcortical structures. They include focal-aware seizures, also called simple partial seizures, and focal impaired awareness seizures, also called complex partial seizures. Focal onset motor seizures include atonic, clonic, automatisms, epileptic spasms, myoclonic, hyperkinetic, and tonic seizures.

Focal onset nonmotor seizures are also classified based on the earliest presenting symptom: autonomic dysfunction involving GI changes, temperature changes, sexual arousal, palpitations and piloerection, behavioral arrest, cognitive dysfunction, emotional dysfunction, and sensory dysfunction.

Unknown-onset seizures – These seizures are classified based on ambiguity in their origins. They can be motor or nonmotor. Unknown motor seizures include epileptic spasms and tonic-clonic seizures. Unknown-onset nonmotor seizures include behavior arrest.

Emergency care

1. Position the patient in the left lateral position.
2. Protect the patient from potential falls.
3. Do a primary survey.
4. Suction the airway if necessary and use airway devices to keep airway patent.
5. Use BVM ventilation if needed.
6. Transport to the ER.

Stroke

Ischemic stroke – This makes up 80% of stroke cases. Causes are lacunar infarcts in the cerebral circulation, cardioembolism, atherosclerosis of large vessels, and cryptogenic infarcts.

Hemorrhagic stroke – This makes up 20% of all stroke cases. These strokes include intracerebral hemorrhage and subarachnoid hemorrhage.

Causes/risk factors – In ischemic stroke, modifiable risk factors are atherosclerosis, diabetes mellitus, dyslipidemia, cigarette smoking, animal obesity, alcoholism, psychosocial stress, hypercoagulability, and vasculitis. Nonmodifiable risk factors are a history of stroke, family history of stroke, race, age, and sex.
In hemorrhagic stroke, the etiology of subarachnoid hemorrhage includes trauma to the head and ruptured aneurysms. Risk factors for intracerebral hemorrhage are rupture of atherosclerotic arteries, congenital aneurysms, vascular malformations, blood dyscrasia, vasculitis, excessive anticoagulation, and hemorrhagic infarction.

Clinical features – These include altered sensorium, hypertension, features of end-organ damage, and raised ICP.

Emergency care

1. Do a primary assessment: airway, breathing, circulation, and drugs.
2. Transport the patient to the nearest stroke center or ER unit.
3. Management is supportive and occurs in a stroke center. It includes:
    a. Acute resuscitation
    b. Antihypertensive therapy in severe hypertension and end-organ dysfunction
    c. Antiplatelet therapy for ischemic stroke
    d. Surgical interventions for hemorrhagic strokes
    e. Treatment of hyperthermia, hyperglycemia/hypoglycemia
    f. Physiotherapy

Syncope

This is a temporary and sudden loss of consciousness caused by a sudden drop in blood supply to the brain, usually due to orthostatic hypotension.

Causes – Noncardiac causes include dehydration, heatstroke, orthostatic hypotension, diabetes, high altitude, Parkinson's, antihypertensives, and migraine. A vasovagal response can be triggered by micturition, coughing, defecations, swallowing, and phlebotomy. Cardiac causes include arrhythmia, hypertension, aortic dissection, and cardiomyopathy.

Emergency care

Place the patient in a supine position and give oxygen via BVM or non-rebreather mask.

Immunologic Emergencies

Anaphylaxis

Atopic and allergic reactions are all Type 1 hypersensitivity reactions, which are mediated by IgE immune response. Examples of atopic disorders are atopic dermatitis, urticaria, angioedema, latex allergies, allergic rhinitis, and others.

Anaphylaxis

This is an acute and life-threatening form of IgE-mediated hypersensitivity reaction.

Causes – These include allergens in insulin, beta-lactam antibiotics, streptokinase, allergens in foods (nuts, eggs and seafood), latex, animal venom, and blood transfusions.

Clinical features – These include urticaria, flushing, pruritus, rhinorrhea, diarrhea, dizziness, syncope, and wheezing. More serious complications like shock, angioedema, cyanosis, and respiratory failure.

Treatment – This includes IV epinephrine and acute resuscitation with IV fluids. Oxygen and vasopressors are used where necessary. Oral antihistamines are given for pruritus, and nebulized beta-agonists are given for respiratory symptoms.

Emergency care

Primary survey

1. Airway – Assess vocal cords. Use airway devices if necessary and commence BVM ventilation.
2. Breathing – Assess the respiratory rate and quality of respiration.

3. Circulation – Check pulse and blood pressure. Give a vasopressor to increase blood pressure if necessary.

Secondary survey

1. Clinical history and examination – History of allergies include the time of exposure and form of exposure. History of interventions.
2. Assess vital signs.
3. Give preloaded epinephrine if the patient has not already taken some.
4. Reassess vital signs and record.
5. Patients should not be given epinephrine if there are no signs of hypotension or respiratory distress.

Toxicology and Poisonings

Organophosphates

Examples – Chlorpyrifos, malathion, parathion, diazinon, Dursban, and fenthion.

Clinical features – Acute presentations are a result of stimulation of muscarinic receptors, lacrimation, salivation, diarrhea, emesis, bronchospasm, bradycardia, bronchorrhea, miosis, muscle weakness, and muscle fasciculations. Late-onset features include weakness of respiratory muscles and axonal neuropathy.

Treatment

1. Acute resuscitation
2. Decontamination when necessary
3. IV atropine for respiratory symptoms
4. Pralidoxime for neuromuscular symptoms
5. Benzodiazepines for seizures

Acids and alkalis

Sources – Toilet cleaners and liquid or solid drain cleaners. Caustic poisoning in children is often accidental ingestion, while in adults it is often intentional.

Clinical features – Symptoms of initial poisoning are dysphagia and drooling. In severe poisoning, patients experience vomiting and upper GI bleeding. If the airway is burned, patients present with stridor and cough. Complications like esophageal and gastric perforation are very likely. Esophageal strictures are late-onset complications.

Principles of treatment
Treatment is supportive with IV fluids and monitoring of metabolic and hematologic profiles. Patients with perforation are managed with IV antibiotics and surgery.

Gastric emptying is contraindicated due to the risk of re-exposing the upper GI tract to the agent. The use of activated charcoal is contraindicated due to the risk of disrupting endoscopy. Insertion of gastrointestinal tubes is contraindicated, as is the use of acids or alkalis to neutralize the agent.

Carbon monoxide
Sources – Fumes from automobiles, kerosene heaters, charcoal or woodstoves, water heaters, furnaces, and gas heaters.

Clinical features – As a result of hypoxia, patients suffer nausea, headaches, dizziness, impaired judgment, inability to concentrate, chest pain, and difficulty breathing. In severe poisoning, patients experience seizures and syncope. Death ensues from severe hypoxia.

Treatment – Supplemental 100% oxygen, or hyperbaric oxygen that displaces carbon dioxide from the red blood cells.

Cyanide
Source – Bitter almond oil, poorly processed cassava products, sodium nitroprusside, wild cherry syrup, prussic acid, hydrocyanic acid, and potassium cyanide.

Clinical features – These include drowsiness, headaches, disorientation, dizziness, and tachycardia. In severe cases, patients experience hypotension, seizures, and coma. The presence of bright red mucosal surfaces requires rapid intervention due to the high risk of mortality. Cyanide is lethal.

Treatment – Supplemental 100% oxygen, inhalational amyl nitrate, and sodium thiosulfate.

Drug interactions
Most likely occur with alternative therapies. Common drugs implicated in interactions are:

1. Warfarin – Aspirin, antacids, acetaminophen, fluconazole, ibuprofen, OTC cold medications, amiodarone, and others. Implicated complementary drugs include ginkgo biloba, St John's wort, green tea, vitamin E, ginseng, garlic, and coenzyme Q10.
2. Fluoxetine and phenelzine – Serotonin syndrome.
3. Quinidine and digoxin – Digoxin toxicity.
4. Sildenafil and nitrates – Massive hypotension.
5. Clonidine and propranolol – Hypertension.
6. Ciprofloxacin and theophylline – Theophylline toxicity.
7. Methotrexate and probenecid – Methotrexate poisoning.

Overdose and ingestions

<u>**Acetaminophen overdose**</u>
Clinical features – These include nausea, vomiting, abdominal cramps, hepatomegaly, pancreatitis, and hepatic failure.

Treatment
1. Use of activated charcoal within four hours of ingestion.
2. Use of the antidote N-acetylcysteine within eight hours of ingestion.
3. Supportive management of gastroenteritis and liver failure.
4. Liver transplantation may be needed in rapidly progressive liver failure.

<u>**Aspirin poisoning**</u>
Clinical features – Nausea, vomiting, hyperventilation, and tinnitus. Patients also present with confusion, fever, seizure, and restlessness. In severe cases, patients can deteriorate to acute renal failure, rhabdomyolysis, and respiratory failure.

Treatment
1. Activated charcoal if ingested within four hours of presentation
2. Fluid and electrolyte replacement
3. Alkaline diuresis with sodium bicarbonate
4. Hemodialysis in severe poisoning

Opioid overdose

Clinical features – These include respiratory depression, apnea, miosis, hypotension, delirium, bradycardia, hypothermia, and urinary retention.

Treatment

1. Acute resuscitation
2. Mechanical ventilation
3. IV naloxone

Iron poisoning

A common cause of accidental poisoning in children.

Clinical features – Acute onset presentation includes nausea, hematemesis, diarrhea, and abdominal cramps. Late-onset presentation includes shock, metabolic acidosis, seizures, and coagulopathy. Complications are liver failure and gastric outlet obstruction.

Treatment – Whole-bowel irrigation with polyethylene glycol, an osmotic laxative, and use of IV deferoxamine in severe poisoning.

Anxiolytic poisoning

Clinical features – These include depressed superficial reflexes, ataxia, impaired coordination, nystagmus, confusion, respiratory depression, and death.

Treatment – Supportive with mechanical ventilation. Use of flumazenil, a benzodiazepine receptor antagonist.

Substance abuse

1. Substance-induced disorders – Intoxication, overdose, withdrawal, and substance-related psychiatric disorders
2. Substance abuse disorders – Addiction, tolerance, physical and psychological dependence

Withdrawal syndrome

Opioids

Clinical features – These include severe physical dependence. Symptoms, which are not usually fatal, include anxiety, tachypnea, diaphoresis, lacrimation, yawning, rhinorrhea, diarrhea, anorexia, tremors, fever, tachycardia, hypertension, and stomach cramps.

Treatment – Symptomatic management and treatment with methadone, clonidine, and naltrexone.

Alcohol

Clinical features – Mild symptoms include headaches, tremors, weakness, diaphoresis, tachycardia, hypertension, seizures, gastrointestinal symptoms and hyperreflexia. Symptoms progress to involve alcoholic hallucinosis characterized by visual and auditory hallucinations and nightmares. Delirium tremens is a late-onset symptom characterized by increasing anxiety, depression, sweating, disorientation, autonomic features, altered personality, tachycardia and hyperthermia. Alcoholic withdrawal symptoms are fatal.

Treatment – Supportive treatment of symptoms, including IV fluids, nutrition, treatment of hyperthermia and use of benzodiazepines for sedation.

Anxiolytics

Clinical features – Withdrawal symptoms of benzodiazepines are not life-threatening. However, withdrawal from barbiturates can mimic life-threatening symptoms similar to delirium tremens.

Features of benzodiazepine withdrawal are tachycardia, tachypnea, hyperpyrexia, and seizures. Features of barbiturate withdrawal include restlessness, increasing anxiety, hyperreflexia, muscle weakness, delirium, insomnia, visual and auditory hallucinations, seizures (which can progress to status epilepticus), and death.

Treatment – Supportive management of symptoms in the ICU. Use of long-acting benzodiazepines.

Nicotine

Nicotine causes strong physical dependence.

Clinical features – Features are irritability, difficulty concentrating, anxiety, depression, aviation, insomnia, hunger, GI disturbances, headaches, and weight gain.

Treatment – Bupropion SR, varenicline, and nicotine replacement therapy.

Cannabis

Withdrawal symptoms of cannabis are generally mild since they do not produce profound physical dependence. Dependence is more psychological.

Clinical features – These include insomnia, nausea, irritability, anorexia, and depression.

Treatment – Not often needed. In severe cases, supportive management is done.

Gastrointestinal Emergencies

Acute abdomen

Appendicitis
Inflammation of the vermiform appendix.

Causes – Obstruction by a hypertrophied lymphoid tissue, fecalith, worms, or foreign bodies.

Clinical features – Fever, anorexia and vomiting, abdominal pain, rebound tenderness, psoas sign, obturator sign, and Rovsing's sign.

Treatment – Appendectomy, which must be done quickly to reduce the risk of perforation and peritonitis.

Upper GI bleeding
Causes – The most common cause is a duodenal ulcer, followed by esophageal varices. Other causes are erosive gastritis, gastric ulcers, Mallory-Weiss tears, arteriovenous malformations, erosive esophagitis, hemobilia, tumors of the gastrointestinal stromal, and angioma.

Clinical features – These include hematemesis, melena stools, and hematochezia in severe cases. Patients can also present with signs of hypovolemic shock, tachycardia, pallor, hypotension, and syncope.

Treatment – Acute resuscitation with IV fluids and oxygen where indicated for patients with shock. Definitive treatment depends on the cause.

Lower GI bleeding
Causes – These include anal fissures, angiodysplasia, colorectal cancer, internal hemorrhoids, colonic polyps, Crohn's disease, and ulcerative colitis.

Clinical features – These include hematochezia, constipation, diarrhea, abdominal cramps, intestinal bloating, and symptoms of hypovolemic shock.

Treatment – Acute resuscitation for those in cardiovascular collapse. Treatment of the underlying cause.

Cholecystitis

Causes – The most common cause is cholelithiasis. Impacted gallstones cause bile stasis, inflammation of the mucosa of the gallbladder, and superseding bacterial infection. If left untreated, there is a high risk of necrosis and gallbladder perforation. Causes of acalculous cholecystitis include total parenteral nutrition, prolonged fasting, critical illness, vasculitis, and immune deficiency. This form of cholecystitis is thought to be caused by bile stasis, infection, and ischemia.

Clinical features – These include biliary colic, characterized by right hypochondrial pain; tenderness in the right hypochondrium, which can be elicited by the Murphy sign; low-grade fever; and nonspecific symptoms like nausea, anorexia, malaise, and vomiting. Complications include perforation, peritonitis, and gallstone pancreatitis.

Treatment – Supportive treatment of symptoms—IV fluids, antibiotics, and analgesia. The definite treatment is cholecystectomy.

Cirrhosis

The advanced stage of hepatic fibrosis is characterized by regenerative nodules of hepatic tissue that are surrounded by fibrotic tissue.

Causes – These include alcoholic liver disease; non-alcoholic fatty liver disease; chronic hepatitis B and hepatitis C infection; primary sclerosing cholangitis; primary biliary cholangitis; autoimmune hepatitis; and drugs like tolbutamide, amiodarone, isoniazid, methyldopa, and methotrexate.

Clinical features – These include stigmata of chronic liver disease, which include jaundice, ascites, pedal edema, skin atrophy, testicular atrophy, gynecomastia, Dupuytren contracture, parotitis, lanugo hair, finger clubbing, paronychia, caput medusae, xanthelasma, asterixis, pallor, and petechiae rashes.

Complications are a result of decompensated liver failure. They include esophageal varices, rectal varices, caput medusae, hepatic encephalopathy, thromboembolism, portal hypertension, hepatorenal syndrome, hepatopulmonary syndrome, spontaneous bacterial peritonitis, and others.

Treatment – The definite treatment is a liver transplant. Supportive management of symptoms includes reduced protein intake, bowel sterilization, use of motility drugs like Dulcolax to prevent constipation, and restriction of the use of sedatives in patients with decompensated liver failure. Transjugular intrahepatic portosystemic shunts are used in patients with portal hypertension.

Diverticulitis

Causes/risk factors – These include red meat, cytomegalovirus infection, and previous history of diverticulitis.

Clinical features – Pain in the left lower quadrant of the abdomen. The pain can also be in the right lower quadrant or suprapubic area. In some patients, there are palpable masses in the sigmoid colon. Other features are fever, nausea, and urinary frequency or urgency. Complications are peritonitis, bowel obstruction, and fistula, which may present as fecaluria, pneumonitis, infection of the abdominal wall, or passage of feculent vaginal discharge.

Treatment – Antibiotic therapy with empiric antibiotics for anaerobic and aerobic bacterial infection, percutaneous drainage of the abscess, and surgery for patients with peritonitis or intestinal obstruction.

Esophageal varices

Causes – Portal hypertension from decompensated liver failure. In this condition, portal pressure is higher than that in the inferior vena cava. This causes shunting of blood via venous collateral in the esophagus, fundus of the stomach, and rectum. These varices have a risk of rupturing and causing severe upper GI bleeding.

Clinical features – Features of upper GI bleeding; hematemesis, which is painless, severe, and sudden. Complications include hypovolemic shock and hepatic encephalopathy.

Treatment

1. Immediate resuscitation: airway, IV fluids, blood products and vasopressors where indicated
2. Endoscopic banding
3. Sclerotherapy
4. Use of IV octreotide
5. Mechanical compression with Sengstaken-Blakemore tube
6. Transjugular intrahepatic portosystemic shunts for persistent bleeding

Esophagitis

Causes – Eosinophilic esophagitis is caused by an immune response to antigens in food. Gastroesophageal reflux disease is caused by incompetence of the lower esophageal sphincter and regurgitation of the gastric contents into the lower esophagus.

Risk factors that lower the competence of the lower esophageal sphincters are obesity; alcohol; tobacco; fatty foods; and drugs like progesterone, calcium channel blocker, nitrates, antihistamines, tricyclic antidepressants, and anticholinergics.

Clinical features – These include heartburn, epigastric pain, dyspepsia, dysphagia, odynophagia, and, in patients with chronic aspiration, cough and wheezing. Complications of esophagitis are esophageal strictures, esophageal ulcers, Barrett's esophagus, and esophageal adenocarcinoma.

Treatment

1. Obese patients are encouraged to lose weight.
2. Alcohol consumption and cigarette smoking are stopped, and implicated drugs are stopped or replaced with others.
3. The head of the bed is elevated in the semi-Fowler's position, especially after eating.
4. Patients are advised to stop eating at least three hours before going to bed.
5. Fatty foods are also avoided.
6. Drug therapy is commenced: proton pump inhibitors, H2 receptor blockers, and antacids to reduce the acidic content of the stomach.

Foreign bodies

Esophageal – The most common cause is impacted food that is not properly chewed, steaks, fishbones, and hot dogs. Infants and toddlers have a high risk of choking on small, round foods like candy, peas, peanuts, and pieces of cut fruits and vegetables. Complications include perforation of the esophagus and obstruction.

Gastric – Gastric bezoars are undigested materials that accumulate in the stomach to form stone-like materials. Examples are phytobezoars, which are made from undigested fruit and vegetable seeds, peels, or fiber; diospyrobezoars, made from the accumulation of persimmon fruit; trichobezoars, made of hair; lactobezoars, made of milk protein; and pharmacobezoars, made of drugs. Bezoars can also be made of inorganic substances like Styrofoam cups and tissue paper. Risk factors include patients with psychiatric disorders, gastric bypass surgery, infants, elderly patients, diabetes mellitus, and hypochlorhydria.

Intestinal – This includes foreign objects in the esophagus and stomach that migrate to the intestine and body packing or body stuffing with heroin or cocaine and other substances.

Rectal – This includes swallowed foreign bodies, fecaliths, gallstones, vaginal pessaries, surgical materials, sex toys, urinary calculi, and drug packets.

Gastritis

Causes – Erosive gastritis is caused by alcohol, NSAIDs, radiation, viral infection, direct trauma, stress and Crohn's disease. Nonerosive gastritis is caused by H pylori infection.

Clinical features – These include anorexia, dyspepsia, nausea, and vomiting. In severe cases, there is hematemesis, the passage of melena stools, or hematochezia.

Treatment – Patients with upper GI bleeding are resuscitated with IV fluids and supplemental oxygen where needed. Bleeding is controlled endoscopically.

For all patients with gastritis, acid suppression drugs, like proton pump inhibitors, antacids and H2 receptor antagonists, are used.

For H pylori infection, antibiotics are used. Triple therapy includes proton pump inhibitors, amoxicillin or metronidazole, and clarithromycin. Quadruple therapy includes proton pump inhibitors, metronidazole, tetracycline, and bismuth subsalicylate.

Gastroenteritis

Causes – Infectious gastroenteritis is caused by viral, bacterial, protozoal, or fungal infections. The most implicated organisms in viral gastroenteritis are rotavirus and norovirus. The most implicated organisms in bacterial gastroenteritis are Clostridium difficile, salmonella, shigella, E. coli, and campylobacter. Implicated organisms in parasitic gastroenteritis are giardia, cryptosporidium, and Entamoeba histolytica.

Clinical features – These include nausea, anorexia, vomiting, diarrhea, and abdominal cramps. Diarrhea may be bloody or mucoid. Patients may also experience specific symptoms like malaise and myalgia. Complications include dehydration, metabolic alkalosis, hypovolemic shock, hemolytic uremic syndrome, metabolic acidosis, and electrolyte derangement.

Treatment – Fluid resuscitation with oral or IV fluids. Antibiotics for bacterial and parasitic infections. Antidiarrheal agents in older patients after ruling out C. difficile and E. coli O157:H7 infection.

Hepatitis

Causes – Infectious causes include hepatitis A, B, C, D, and E viruses; cytomegalovirus; yellow fever; infectious mononucleosis; amebiasis; malaria; and schistosomiasis. Other causes include alcohol, hypercholesterolemia, autoimmune disorders, genetic diseases of the liver, and infiltrative diseases like amyloidosis and sarcoidosis.

Clinical features – This depends on the cause. Examples are jaundice, pruritus, pale stools, dark-colored urine, fever, malaise, and anorexia. Patients may also present with stigmata of chronic liver disease.

Treatment

1. Treatment of underlying cause. Hepatitis A and E infections are often short lived and require no antibiotic treatment, just supportive management of symptoms. Hepatitis B infection is chronic and has no treatment. It is, however, preventable with a vaccine. Hepatitis C infection is treatable with direct-acting antivirals like telaprevir, simeprevir, sofosbuvir, dasabuvir, ombitasvir, and daclatasvir.
2. Removal of risk factors (alcohol, offending drugs) and use of antilipids for fatty liver disease.
3. Supportive management, including nutrition, IV fluids for rehydration, cholestyramine for pruritus, and management of complications in patients with chronic liver disease.

Hernia

Inguinal hernia – A direct inguinal hernia bypasses the inguinal canal and pushes directly out from the external abdominal wall. The indirect inguinal canal transverse the inguinal ring and enters the inguinal canal. Causes of an inguinal hernia include increased intra-abdominal pressure (coughing, constipation and lifting of heavy objects).

Umbilical hernia – Protrusions through the umbilical canal are mostly congenital. Secondary causes are pregnancy, obesity, and ascites.

Epigastric hernia – Protrusion through a defect in the linea alba.

Femoral hernia – Bulging of a loop of the femoral artery through the femoral canal below the inguinal ligament. The mass is pulsatile.

Clinical features – The presence of a bulging mass that may or may not be reducible. If the mass is strangulated or incarcerated, patients present to the ER with worsening pain that may be associated with nausea, vomiting, and dehydration. In severe cases, patients present with peritonitis.

Treatment – All hernias are treated via surgical repair. Patients who present to the ER with strangulated or incarcerated hernias must be treated via emergency surgical repair to reduce the risk of perforation.

Inflammatory bowel disease

Crohn's disease

Chronic inflammation of the ileum and colon.

Clinical features – These include chronic diarrhea with fever, anorexia, abdominal pain, and weight loss. On examination, there is tenderness of the abdomen with a palpable mass. In complicated cases, patients present with an acute abdomen. Complications include malabsorption syndromes, colorectal cancer, and toxic megacolon. Children may present with extraintestinal symptoms like fever of unknown origin, anemia, arthritis, and growth retardation.

Ulcerative colitis

Chronic inflammation of the colonic mucosa.

Clinical features – These include episodes of bloody diarrhea with asymptomatic episodes. Patients can also have episodes of constipation that alternate with episodes of diarrhea. Patients may also experience discharge of bloody mucus in between bowel movements. Nonspecific symptoms include fever, malaise, anorexia, anemia, and weight loss. Extraintestinal symptoms include joint and skin disorders.

Intussusception

Causes – Mostly idiopathic. Risk is higher in young children and males, during the peak season of viral enteritis. Other risk factors include cystic fibrosis, Merkel's diverticulum, gastrointestinal polyps, and lymphoma.

Clinical features – Colicky abdominal pain is the earliest symptom. Other symptoms are lethargy, dehydration, and passage of jelly-like stool. In complicated cases, the patient presents with intestinal obstruction, or perforation and peritonitis.

Treatment – Air enema for reduction of the bowel. Surgical interventions for failed air enemas.

Obstructions

Causes – The most common causes include hernias, tumors, and adhesions. Other causes are foreign body impaction, volvulus, fecal impaction, and intussusception.

Clinical features – These include abdominal cramps and vomiting. Patients with complete obstruction experience obstipation, while patients with partial obstruction experience diarrhea. Bowel sounds are hyperactive. Absent bowel sounds indicate peritonitis.

In complicated cases, patients present with shock. Obstructions of the large intestine are milder than obstructions of the small intestine. Patients present with constipation, vomiting, and abdominal cramps. A mass may be palpable.

Treatment
This is a surgical emergency. Treatment modalities include:

1. Placing the patient on NPO.
2. Nasogastric suction.
3. Fluid and electrolyte replacement via IV fluids.
4. Measurement of fluid input and output (via urethral catheter).
5. IV antibiotics.
6. Definitive treatment is surgical exploration, resection and anastomosis where appropriate.

Pancreatitis
Causes – The most common causes are alcoholism and gallstones. Other causes are viral infections with mumps, cytomegalovirus and coxsackievirus B, metabolic causes like hypercalcemia, hypertriglyceridemia, trauma, pancreatic cancer, and others.

Clinical features – These include upper abdominal pain, nausea, vomiting, hypotension, and fever. Significant findings are Cullen's and Turner's signs. In complicated cases, patients have paralytic ileus, peritonitis, infection, and sepsis with multiple organ dysfunction.

Treatment – Supportive management of dehydration, hypoglycemia, infections, and pain. Patients need adequate nutrition via an enteral feeding tube. Adequate pain relief.

Ulcers
Causes – These include H. pylori infection, NSAIDs, cigarette smoking, alcohol, and family history.

Clinical features – Patients with gastric ulcers experience epigastric pain that is worsened by eating. Other symptoms include nausea, vomiting, and bloating. Patients with duodenal ulcers experience epigastric pain that is relieved by food and recurs two to three hours after eating. Nocturnal pain that rouses the patient from sleep is seen in duodenal ulcers. Complications include upper GI bleeding, perforation, peritonitis, gastric outlet syndrome, and an increased risk for stomach cancer.

Infection Control and Personal Protection

Safety guidelines

Handwashing
Handwashing with soap and water prevents the transmission of droplets and air-borne diseases. Wash hands before coming into contact with broken skin, after handling patients, and after coming into contact with patients' environments.

Eye protection
Eye shields are used when there is a potential for eye injury when extracting patients from vehicles. They are also worn when there is a risk of splashing bodily fluids onto the face.

Gloves
Gloves must be worn before coming into contact with all patients and when handling bodily fluids. They must be changed before contact with a new patient.

Gowns
Gowns are used to protect the body from splashes from bodily fluids.

Masks
Masks are used to protect EMTs both from splashes of bodily fluids and from aerosols and droplets.

Protection from hazmat incidents

Hazmat incidents require specialized suits. All EMTs must be educated on how to use the self-contained breathing apparatus in their suit. Usually, specialized teams are deployed to hazmat scenes, after which EMTs can proceed to provide emergency services to patients. EMTs who are not trained to function as response teams to hazmat incidents can work only in the cold zone.

Endocrine Emergencies

Diabetic ketoacidosis

Pathophysiology – Marked hyperglycemia causes osmotic diuresis and dehydration. Also, insulin deficiency causes ketogenesis from fatty acids and proteins. Ketonemia causes metabolic acidosis and worsens dehydration. Osmotic diuresis causes the depletion of sodium and potassium ions.

Causes – These include physiologic stress from acute infections (UTIs and pneumonia), stroke, pancreatitis, myocardial infarction, trauma, and drugs (thiazide, sympathomimetic, and corticosteroids).

Clinical features – These include severe dehydration, polyuria, polydipsia, restlessness, personality change, altered consciousness, ketone breath, vomiting, abdominal pain, and hyperglycemic coma.

Emergency care

1. Conduct a primary survey and assessment.
2. Call for assistance in ALS.
3. Monitor and record vital signs.
4. Transport patient quickly.

Hypoglycemia

Pathophysiology – Symptomatic hypoglycemia is often caused by insulin injections and use of oral antidiabetic drugs. Physiologic hypoglycemia can be grouped into fasting, reactive insulin-mediated, noninsulin-mediated, drug-induced, and nondrug-induced.

Clinical features – These include nausea, anxiety, sweating, shaking, hunger, paresthesia palpitations, confusion, headaches, seizures, double vision, and coma.

Emergency care

1. Do a primary survey.
2. Do a secondary survey and take a patient history.
3. Administer oral glucose solution if the patient can tolerate oral fluids.
4. Transport to the ER.

Genitourinary Emergencies

Foreign bodies

Causes – These include iatrogenic, sexual abuse, assault, self-insertion in children, psychiatric disorders or fetish behaviors, and migration from other sites.

Clinical features – Adults are more likely to present late due to embarrassment. Patients often present with pain, urinary tract infection, and hematuria. Strictures are likely complications.

Treatment – Instrumental or surgical removal of the object.

Pyelonephritis

Causes – Most often caused by enteric gram-negative bacteria. Risk factors include female sex, obstructive uropathy, urethral catheterization, chronic constipation, and menopause.

Clinical features – Patients with uncomplicated cases present with fever, flank/lower abdominal pain, anorexia, nausea, vomiting, dysuria, and hematuria. Patients with complicated cases present with symptoms of acute kidney injury (oliguria, hypertension, and fluid retention).

Treatment

1. Treatment with empiric IV antibiotics until results of bacterial culture and sensitivity are obtained
2. Supportive management of pain and other symptoms
3. Management of acute kidney injury in patients who present with it
4. Treatment of the underlying cause and elimination of risk factors

Epididymitis

Causes – Causes of bacterial epididymitis are chlamydia trachomatis and Neisseria gonorrhea in most males younger than 35. In males who are older than 35, gram-negative coliform bacteria are the most implicated bacteria. These organisms are often seen in patients with obstructive uropathy or retained catheters.

Nonbacterial causes of epididymitis are viruses, like cytomegalovirus, and fungi, like Blastomyces and actinomycetes. Noninfectious causes are trauma and retrograde flow of urine.

Clinical features – Scrotal pain is the cardinal symptom. Other features are fever, nausea, anorexia, and vomiting. Patients also experience irritative urinary symptoms (frequency, urgency, incontinence, dysuria, and hematuria). In complicated cases, patients present with septic shock.

Treatment – Supportive management, such as bed rest; elevation of the scrotum; and analgesia. Antibiotic therapy.

Orchitis

Causes – Infections that are localized to just the testes are mainly caused by viruses (mumps). Other causes are leprosy, tuberculosis, varicella-zoster infection, coxsackievirus infection, and congenital syphilis.

Clinical features – These include testicular pain, edema, and induration. Patients may also experience systemic symptoms, like fever, nausea, vomiting, and myalgia. On testicular examination, there is tenderness and induration of the testes and scrotal skin.

Treatment – Antibiotics for bacterial causes. Supportive measures with analgesia for viral causes.

Priapism

Causes – These include drugs used to treat erectile dysfunction (sildenafil, phentolamine, alprostadil and papaverine); recreational drugs, like cocaine and amphetamines; hematologic disorders, like leukemia, sickle cell anemia, and lymphoma; advanced prostate cancer; beta-blockers; antipsychotics; anticoagulants; oral hypoglycemic agents; and lithium.

Clinical features – Persistent, painful, and abnormal erection without sexual desire.

Treatment

Ischemic priapism

1. Aspiration of blood from the corpora cavernosa with a nonheparinized syringe.
2. Intracavernous injection of phenylephrine.
3. Irrigation with normal saline.
4. Creation of a surgical shunt for cases unresponsive to the above listed.
5. For patients with sickle cell anemia, management of vaso-occlusive crisis is required.

Nonischemic priapism

1. Analgesia and cold compression with ice packs.
2. For cases unresponsive to the above, surgery is required.

Renal calculi

Causes/risk factors – Risk factors for calcium calculi are hypercalciuria from hypocitraturia, renal tubular acidosis, hyperoxaluria, primary hyperparathyroidism, vitamin D poisoning, hyperthyroidism, and multiple myeloma. Other causes of calcium calculi are vitamin C hypervitaminosis and hyperuricosuria. Cystine calculi are caused by cystinuria, while magnesium ammonium phosphate calculi are caused by chronic urinary tract infections.

Clinical features – Renal colic with nausea and vomiting. Patients may present with symptoms of urinary tract infection and/or symptoms of obstructive uropathy.

Testicular torsion

Cause – Anomalies in the development of the tunica vaginalis and spermatic cord cause incomplete fixation of the testis to the tunica vaginalis. Torsion is common in males ages 12 to 18 years with such anomalies. It is most likely to occur in the left testis.

Clinical features – Severe testicular pain accompanied by nausea and vomiting. In inspection, the testes are tender, swollen, and indurated. They may be elevated and horizontal. Cremasteric reflex on the affected testes is absent.

Treatment – Analgesia for prompt relief. Manual detorsion. Emergency surgery for failed detorsion.

Bladder trauma

Causes – Blunt or penetrating trauma to the pelvis, perineum, or suprapubic region of the abdomen. Blunt trauma is the most common cause following a vehicle crash, an external blow to the abdomen, or a fall. Patients are also likely to have pelvic fractures.

The bladder can also be injured during pelvic surgeries, especially abdominal hysterectomy; excision of a pelvic mass; and caesarean section. Risks increase when there is fibrosis from surgery or radiation exposure and when the tumor to be excised is extensive.

Clinical features – These include suprapubic pain, urine retention and hematuria. Patients may also present with abdominal distension, peritonitis, and hypovolemic shock. Complications are urine ascites, persistent hematuria, infections and sepsis, incontinence, and formation of a fistula.

Treatment – Drainage with a catheter. Exploration and surgical repair.

Urinary retention

Causes – These include bladder outlet obstruction; impaired contractility of the bladder; anticholinergics; fecal impaction; and, in patients with neurogenic bladder, multiple sclerosis, diabetes, and Parkinson's.

Clinical features – These include a feeling of incomplete voiding, frequency, suprapubic swelling, and suprapubic pain. In complicated cases, patients present with symptoms of urinary tract infections and/or obstructive uropathy.

Treatment – Prompt relief of symptoms via urethral/suprapubic catheterization. Treatment of underlying cause.

Gynecologic Emergencies

Bleeding/dysfunction

Dysfunctional uterine bleeding is caused by ovulatory disorders.

Causes – Causes of anovulatory abnormal uterine bleeding include structural causes of hypothalamic dysfunction (hypothalamic tumors, irradiation, traumatic brain injury), genetic disorders affecting the hypothalamus, and infiltrative disorders.

Functional causes of hypothalamic dysfunction include eating disorders; depression; drugs, like cocaine; malnutrition;; obesity; excessive exercise; diets; food fads; and chronic diseases. Other causes include disorders of the pituitary and ovaries and endocrine abnormalities.

Causes of ovulatory abnormal uterine bleeding include endometriosis, polycystic ovarian syndrome, and inadequate stimulation of the endometrium with progesterone.

Clinical features – Polymenorrhea, which is a menstrual cycle that is less than 21 days; menorrhagia, which is bleeding that lasts for more than 7 days; metrorrhagia, which is bleeding in between periods; and menometrorrhagia, which is increased bleeding and bleeding in between periods. Patients may also experience painful menstruation and premenstrual symptoms.

Treatment – Acute resuscitation in women with active bleeding and hypovolemic shock. Correction of iron-deficiency anemia. Treatment of underlying cause.

Foreign bodies

Causes – In children, the most common foreign bodies are fibrous threads and materials from clothing or carpets. Also, children may insert crayons and smaller objects into themselves out of curiosity. Larger objects are often a sign of sexual abuse. In teenagers and adults, objects include tampons, broken condoms, or sex toys. Some objects are placed during sexual abuse.

Clinical features – The most common symptoms are foul-smelling vaginal discharge and vaginal bleeding. Less common symptoms are dysuria and hematuria. Foreign bodies can perforate the vagina and cause sepsis. Chronic retention of foreign bodies can lead to the formation of a fistula.

Treatment – Extraction of the object after thorough visualization via cervical and rectal examination. Some objects can be extracted with a speculum, while other objects will require surgical extraction under regional anesthesia.

Hemorrhage

Causes – In adults, causes include ovulatory disorders, like abnormal uterine bleeding, polycystic ovarian syndrome and functional ovarian cysts; inflammatory conditions, like cervicitis; vaginitis; a foreign body in the reproductive tract; endocrine disorders, like hypothyroidism and hyperprolactinemia; coagulation disorders; use of contraceptives, like intrauterine devices or oral contraceptives; depot medroxyprogesterone and hormone replacement therapy; and cancers of the uterus, cervix, and vagina.

In children, causes are precocious puberty, maternal estrogens, urethral prolapse, trauma, sexual abuse, vaginal warts, cervical tumors, exposure to diethylstilbestrol, and foreign bodies in the vagina or cervix.

Treatment – Acute resuscitation for patients with hypotension or hypovolemic shock. Patients are resuscitated with IV fluids, vasopressors, blood products, and supplemental oxygen as indicated. Correction of iron-deficiency anemia. Treatment of underlying cause.

Vaginitis

Causes – In children, the most common cause is infection by flora in the gastrointestinal tract due to improper wiping after urination and poor perineal hygiene. Other causes are foreign bodies in the vagina; certain soaps and bubble baths; tight, nonbreathable underwear; sexual abuse; and obesity (candida vaginitis).

Common causes in women of reproductive age are:
Bacterial vaginosis – Triggered by the destruction of lactobacillus in vaginal flora and proliferation of opportunistic bacteria. Risk factors are douching, multiple sexual partners, poor hygiene, menstrual blood, and semen. All these reduce the acidity of the vagina.

Trichomonas vaginitis – From sexual contact.

Candidal vaginitis – Disruption of the vaginal flora due to use of tight, nonbreathable underwear; obesity; excess heat and humidity; tampons; and chronic use of antibiotics.

In postmenopausal women, the most common cause is atrophic vaginitis caused by decreased estrogen secretion, decreased acidity of the vagina, and disruption of vaginal flora. Other causes are poor perineal hygiene and/or urine and fecal incontinence.

Clinical features – Abnormal vaginal discharge associated with fever, pruritus, dysuria, dyspareunia, and erythema of the labia majora and minora.

Treatment – Symptomatic relief of itching. Treatment of underlying causes.

Cervicitis

Causes – The most common causes are sexually transmitted chlamydia trachomatis and Neisseria gonorrhoeae. Other implicated organisms are trichomonas vaginalis, herpes simplex virus, and mycoplasma. Noninfectious causes include foreign bodies, allergens, chemicals, and the performance of gynecologic procedures.

Clinical features – The most common symptoms are vaginal discharge, dyspareunia, and vaginal bleeding during intercourse or in between periods. Other symptoms are dysmenorrhea, dysuria, and vaginal itching. Significant findings on examination are cervical erythema and edema, oozing of mucopurulent discharge, and cervical friability.

Treatment – Empirical antibiotics based on clinical features, then appropriate antibiotics after retrieving results of microscopy, culture, and sensitivity. Contact tracing and treatment of all sexual partners. Re-evaluation after three months.

Pelvic inflammatory disease

Causes – The most common causes are chlamydia and Neisseria gonorrhoeae. Other microorganisms are mycoplasma, gram-negative bacilli, streptococcus agalactiae, Hemophilus influenzae, and ureaplasma spp. Risk factors include multiple sexual partners, previous history of PID, younger age, douching, and low socioeconomic status.

Complications include hydrosalpinx, Fitz-Hugh-Curtis syndrome, scarring of the fallopian tubes, increased risk of ectopic pregnancies, and tubo ovarian abscess.

Clinical features – Features of vaginitis, cervicitis, and salpingitis.

Treatment – Empirical antibiotic therapy. Screening and treatment of STDs. Contact tracing where appropriate.

Ovarian cyst
Causes – Follicular cysts from Graafian follicles and corpus luteum cysts.

Clinical features – Typically asymptomatic. Patients with ruptured cysts present with lower abdominal pain, features of peritonitis, and hypovolemic shock. In adnexal torsion, patients present with severe lower abdominal pain, nausea, and vomiting. On cervical examination, cervical motion tenderness is positive and the adnexal mass may be palpable.

Treatment – Acute resuscitation for patients with rupture or adnexal torsion. Definite treatment is exploratory laparotomy with cystectomy, salpingectomy, and salpingotomy where indicated.

Sexual assault/battery
This includes rape and inappropriate, nonconsensual touching or holding and the use of threats.

Causes/risk factors – Females are most at risk of sexual assaults.

Clinic features – Victims of rape may present to the ER. Clinical presentations include genital and extragenital injuries, psychological symptoms, features of sexually transmitted diseases, PIDs, and cervicitis. On evaluation, the patient may have PTSD, be pregnant, or have hepatitis or HIV infection.

Evaluation

1. The initial response is to provide safety for patients who present to the ER with their partners, who may be perpetrators of the assault. For rape victims, the goals of evaluation are medical evaluation and prompt treatment of injuries and STDs.
2. Patients should be screened for pregnancy, and appropriate measures must be taken to prevent pregnancy and STDs.
3. Forensic evidence should be collected with the patient's consent to legal intervention.
4. Psychological assessment and support must be provided.
5. Crisis intervention should be recommended to all patients.
6. The sexual assault rape team should be consulted where available.

Obstetric Emergencies

Abruptio placenta

Causes – Risk factors are older maternal age, trauma to the abdomen, hypertension, chorioamnionitis, polyhydramnios, premature rupture of membranes, vasculitis, tobacco use, cocaine use, and maternal thrombotic disorders.

Clinical features – Vaginal bleeding of dark or bright red blood. In patients with retroplacental hemorrhage, there will be no or slight vaginal bleeding. Patients may present with hypovolemic shock in severe bleeding. The uterus is rigid and tender, and there may be signs of fetal distress. Complications include hemodynamic instability, hypovolemic shock, and DIC in the patient. Fetal compromise and fetomaternal transfusion can cause Rh sensitization.

Ectopic pregnancy

Causes/risk factors – These include history of previous ectopic pregnancies, history of pelvic inflammatory diseases, assisted reproduction, intrauterine contraceptive devices, previous tubal surgeries, history of induced abortion, cigarette smoking, and multiple sexual partners.

Clinical features – Presentation in the ER is due to a ruptured ectopic pregnancy. Features include severe lower abdominal pain and vaginal bleeding. To rule out a diagnosis of ruptured ovarian cysts, a pregnancy test is done. Patients are likely to present with features of hypovolemic shock and peritonitis.

Postpartum bleeding

Causes – The most common cause of postpartum hemorrhage is uterine atony. Risk factors for uterine atony are grand multiparity, multiple gestations, polyhydramnios, fetal macrosomia, congenital anomalies, precipitate labor, anesthesia, and chorioamnionitis. Other causes of hemorrhage are uterine rupture, retained products of conception, cervical tears, episiotomies, inversion of the uterus, bleeding disorders and coagulopathies, uterine fibroids, and involution of the placenta.

Clinical features – Vaginal bleeding. Patients rapidly go into hypovolemic shock.

Hyperemesis gravidarum

Causes – Hormonal. Increased levels of estrogens and beta HCG. Morning sickness is a usual occurrence in the first and second trimesters.

Clinical features – In hyperemesis gravidarum, there is severe vomiting that causes dehydration, electrolytes derangement, ketosis, and weight loss. Patients present with features of hypovolemic shock. Complications are fatty degenerative changes in the liver, Wernicke's encephalopathy, and Mallory-Weiss tears.

Neonatal resuscitation

Indications – Birth asphyxia characterized by an Apgar score of less than 7 in the first minute of life.

Principles

Preparation – Identification of perinatal risk factors, like gestational age less than 36 weeks or greater than 41 weeks; operative vaginal delivery; fetal compromise during labor or delivery; emergency caesarean delivery; obstructed labor; and meconium-stained fluid. Preparation also includes the provision of necessary equipment and the presence of at least one person skilled in resuscitation.

The neonate should be given warmth and quickly assessed for an APGAR score. The neonate should also be dried for warmth and stimulation.

Suctioning with a bulb syringe is used for infants with aspiration or obstruction of the airway. The cord should be clamped, and babies who do not require resuscitation must be quickly given to their mother to establish skin-to-skin contact.

Ventilation and oxygenation – For babies who require resuscitation, stimulation is given via flicking the soles or rubbing the back. Suctioning is not used as a form of stimulation. If the APGAR score is low in the next one minute of stimulation, positive-pressure ventilation is administered via bag and mask. The neonate is placed in the appropriate position, and the appropriate cuff is used.

Intubation and chest compression – Infants with heart rates less than 100 bpm should be quickly intubated, and chest compressions should be commenced at the rate of three compressions to one breath. In 60 seconds, a total of 90 compressions and 30 breaths should be given. An assistant is used at this stage.

Drugs – If the heart rate remains below 60 beats per minute, epinephrine is given via an endotracheal tube.

Fluids – If the neonate does not respond to resuscitation, volume expanders, like 0.9% saline, are given, and compression and ventilation are recommenced. Pneumothorax should be ruled out.

Placenta previa

Causes – These include older maternal age, multiple gestation, previous caesarean section or myomectomy, multiparity, smoking, and uterine abnormalities.

Clinical features – Sudden and painless vaginal bleeding. The blood is often bright red. There may be no fetal compromise, even in the face of maternal hemodynamic instability. Apart from antepartum hemorrhage, other complications of placenta previa are prelabor rupture of membranes, fetal malpresentation, intrauterine growth restriction, postpartum hemorrhage, and increased risk of placenta accreta.

Postpartum infection

Causes/risk factors – These include chorioamnionitis, prolonged rupture of membranes, caesarean delivery, prolonged labor, invasive fetal monitoring, frequent cervical examination, anemia, postpartum hemorrhage, bacterial vaginosis, low socioeconomic status, and young maternal age. The most implicated organisms are anaerobes, gram-positive cocci, and gram-negative bacteria. The endometrium is most often infected, although the myometrium and parametrium may also be involved.

Clinical features – These include foul-smelling lochia, fever, lower abdominal pain, uterine tenseness, fever, malaise, and anorexia. The patient may present with features of septic shock.

Preeclampsia, eclampsia, HELLP syndrome

Causes/risk factors – These include nulliparity, multiple gestation, hypertension, older or very young maternal age, obesity, family history of preeclampsia, previous history of preeclampsia, and thrombotic disorders.

Clinical features – These include fluid retention, facial puffiness, excessive weight gain, proteinuria, and hypertension. In severe preeclampsia, patients experience visual disturbances, epigastric pain, severe headaches, confusion, difficulty breathing, and oliguria. In eclampsia, patients have seizures, altered neurologic deficits, and coagulopathies.

Preterm labor

Causes – These include chorioamnionitis, prelabor rupture of membranes, multiple gestations, abnormalities of the fetus, congenital malformations, pyelonephritis, sexually transmitted infections, cervical insufficiency, and previous history of preterm labor.

Threatened/spontaneous abortion

Causes – These include cervical insufficiency, congenital malformations not compatible with life, viral infections (cytomegalovirus, rubella virus, parvovirus, and herpes virus) uterine anomalies, and major trauma to the uterus. Risk factors include older maternal age, substance abuse disorders, cigarette smoking, poorly controlled diabetes mellitus or hypertension, and thyroid disorders.

Clinical features – Vaginal bleeding and cramping abdominal pain. In spontaneous abortion, the cervical os is opened and there may be complete expulsion of the fetus. In patients with threatened abortion, the cervical os is closed. If products of conception are retained, sepsis may set in.

Uterine rupture

Causes – These include overdistension of the uterus, multiple gestations, polyhydramnios, and fetal anomalies. Overstimulation with uterotonics, internal or external fetal version, prolonged obstructed labor, and iatrogenic perforation of the uterus. Risk for rupture increases in women with previous caesarean section, myomectomies, or open maternal-fetal surgery.

Clinical features – These include hemorrhagic shock, persistent vaginal bleeding, fetal bradycardia and variable deceleration, floating fetal head, and severe abdominal pain.

Psychiatric Emergencies

Aggressive/violent behavior

Causes – These include psychotic episodes, substance-use disorder, acute mania, delirium, delusional disorders, schizophrenia, intoxication with alcohol, or recreational drugs. Risk increases when a patient has had a prior history of agitation.

Treatment – Treatment and evaluation should be conducted simultaneously. The principle of management is to ensure the patient's safety and the safety of others by putting the patient in a separate room, using therapeutic communication techniques, and using physical or chemical restraints where necessary.

Anxiety/panic

Generalized anxiety disorder – Patients have an excessive display of worry or anxiety that lasts for days for a minimum of six months. Sources of anxiety are health, social interactions, work, and other life activities. Symptoms include restlessness, agitation, easy fatigability, lack of concentration, insomnia, muscle tension, and others.

Panic disorder – Affected individuals have recurrent and unexpected sudden episodes of panic attacks and unexpected episodes of intense fear that build up quickly. Attacks can be expected or caused by certain triggers. Symptoms include palpitations, sweating, shaking, difficulty in breathing, hyperventilation, feeling of doom, and feelings of things spinning out of control.

Phobia-related disorders – A phobia is an intense fear of specific situations or/and objects. In phobias, the fear is out of magnitude to the danger caused by the object/situation. Symptoms include excessive worry, anxiety, panic, and feeling of impending doom. There are different types of phobias, some of which are fear of spiders, blood, flying, and heights.

Social anxiety disorder – This is also known as social phobia. Affected individuals have a deep fear of social situations. They worry that others may negatively interpret their actions. This leads to embarrassment, worry, and avoidance of social gatherings. Affected people worry that others will find their anxiety-fueled actions or behaviors unacceptable, thereby causing embarrassment. As a result, affected individuals avoid social gatherings.

Separation anxiety disorder – Affected individuals are afraid of being separated from people they are attached to. This is often seen in young children, but it can also be seen in adults. Affected individuals may experience nightmares of separation from their attachment figures. They may also experience physical symptoms when separated or when anticipating a separation.

Bipolar disorder

This disorder is characterized by alternating episodes of mania and depression. However, patients may have a predominance of one or the other. Classification of bipolar disorders includes bipolar I disorder, which is characterized by at least one full-fledged manic episode and usually depressive episodes; bipolar II disorder, which is characterized by major depressive episodes with at least one hypomanic episode and no full-fledged manic episodes; and unspecified bipolar disorder, which has clear bipolar features that do not meet the specific criteria for other bipolar disorders.

Depression

This disorder is characterized by severe and persistent sadness that interferes with function. Classification of depression includes major depressive disorder, which is a persistent depressive disorder that lasts for more than two years even with medication; other specified or unspecified depressive disorder; and classification by etiology, which includes premenstrual dysphoric disorders, depressive disorder due to another medical condition, and substance/medication-induced depressive disorder.

Homicidal ideation

This refers to the contemplation of homicide. Risk factors are personality disorders, psychosis, delirium, and substance-induced disorders. Homicidal ideation also occurs in patients with no psychiatric disorder.

Psychosis

Patients with brief psychotic disorder experience hallucinations, delusions, and other symptoms for at least one day. These symptoms last less than a month. Causes are stressful events, pre-existing personality disorders, and conditions like SLE. Treatment is the same as treatment given for schizophrenia.

Situational crisis

This refers to sudden and stressful situations that disrupt an individual's normal activity. The characteristics of a situational crisis are the presence of a stressful event and the individual's inability to cope with the event and intervention. Examples of situational crises are natural disasters; family disruption; life events, like divorce or losing a child; the death of a loved one; suicide; and economic changes.

Suicidal ideation

This includes completed suicide and attempted suicide.

Completed suicide – This is a suicidal act that results in death.

Attempted suicide – This is a nonfatal but injurious act that is self-directed and intended to result in death. It may or may not cause injury.

Nonsuicidal self-injury (NSSI) – This is a self-inflicted injurious act that is not intended to cause death. The causes of suicidal behavior include depression; other mental disorders, like schizophrenia and bipolar disorder; alcohol and substance abuse; previous suicide attempts; unemployment and economic difficulties; personality disorders; impulsivity; traumatic childhood experiences; family history of suicide; mental disorders; and more.

Environmental Emergencies

Submersion injury

Risk factors for drowning

1. African American, Native American, immigrant children from families with low socioeconomic status
2. Males
3. People with seizure disorders
4. People with long QT syndrome
5. People intoxicated with alcohol or other substances
6. People who participate in dangerous underwater breath-holding activities
7. Pathophysiology – Includes hypoxia, aspiration of fluid and hypothermia

Clinical features – Patients who survive present to the ER with hypothermia, wheezing, altered consciousness, and vomiting.

Treatment – Acute resuscitation for apneic patients. Supportive management via assisted ventilation, antibiotics, provision of warmth, and control of electrolyte derangement.

Frostbite

Causes – Extreme cold at high altitudes.

Clinical features – Freezing and numbing of affected areas. When these areas are warmed, they present with tenderness, edema, erythema, and blisters. In severe cases, affected areas become gangrenous and necrotic. Complications are autoamputation, compartment syndrome, and neuropathy.

Treatment

1. Acute resuscitation of the patient. This includes assessment and stabilization of airway breathing and circulation.
2. Provision of warmth.
3. Rewarming of the affected area.
4. Debriding of the wound and wound care.
5. Amputation where appropriate.

Heat exhaustion and heat stroke

Risk factors – Young athletes, manual laborers, children locked in parked vehicles, and elderly patients.

Clinical features – Patients with heat exhaustion experience headaches, nausea, vomiting, and syncope. Patients often have tachycardia and hypotension. In heatstroke, patients have altered sensorium, delirium, confusion, and ataxia.

Treatment – Treat the patient in a cool environment. Provide fluid and electrolyte replacement. Patients with heatstroke are managed with rapid cooling techniques and supportive measures to treat rhabdomyolysis, DIC, and acute kidney injury.

Electrical injuries

Causes – Home accidents are not as serious and can be due to exposure to naked wires, frayed cords, faulty electrical sockets, and electrical appliances. Severe cases are caused by exposure to high voltages in factories.

Clinical features – These include burns that may be more extensive than the cutaneous presentation; ventricular fibrillation; seizures; muscle fasciculation; respiratory arrest; cardiac arrest, damage to the central and/or peripheral nervous system; and associated injuries, like fractures, dislocations, contusions, lacerations, and blunt injuries to internal organs.

Treatment

1. Acute resuscitation via monitoring of airway, breathing and circulation
2. Fluid resuscitation for severe cases and patients with rhabdomyolysis, acute kidney injury or shock
3. Cardiac monitoring
4. Wound debridement and wound care
5. Tetanus prophylaxis

6. Analgesia
7. Management of associated complications

Burns

Thermal burns – From external heat, such as hot liquids, steam, hot solid objects, and flames, and also from smoke inhalation during fires.

Radiation burns – Examples include sunburn from prolonged sun exposure and prolonged exposure to other forms of ultraviolet rays from tanning beds and exposure to nonsolar radiation, like X-rays.

Chemical burns – From acids; alkalis, like cement and lye; and exposure to other corrosive agents, like mustard gas, cresols, phenols, paint thinner, and gasoline. These agents can penetrate deep into the layers of skin and cause extensive burns over hours.

Electrical burns – Exposure to live wires and consequent electrocution. Electrical burns extend into deeper tissues even in the face of minimum skin injury. Burns can extend to muscles, blood vessels, and nerves.

Classification of burns

First-degree burns – Burns affect only the epidermis.

Second-degree burns – Also called partial-thickness burns. They include superficial partial-thickness burns, which involve the epidermis and the superficial dermis. Healing occurs from the epidermal cells in the hair follicles and sweat glands. Deep partial-thickness burns involve the epidermis and deep dermis. Scarring occurs due to extensive fibrosis. Healing starts only from the hair follicles.

Third-degree burns – Also called full-thickness burns. Necrosis involves the epidermis, dermis, and subcutaneous fat. Healing starts from the periphery of the skin and requires skin grafting for extensive burns.

Acute complications – These include smoke inhalation, hypovolemia, hypothermia, sepsis, paralytic ileus, compartment syndrome, and metabolic derangements.

Late-onset complications – Contractures and keloids.

Management

1. Acute resuscitation
2. Clearing and assessing airway, breathing, and circulation

3. Removal of burned clothing, exposure of burnt skin; decontamination where necessary
4. IV analgesia as needed
5. Fluid resuscitation with Parkland formula
6. Wound cleaning and dressing with appropriate dressing materials
7. Tetanus toxoid injection where necessary
8. Supportive measures for hypothermia, compartment syndrome, nutritional ,and others
9. Prompt referral to the burn center as appropriate

Envenomation Emergencies

Causes – These include snakes, spiders, and aquatic organisms. Snake bites are mostly from rattlesnakes, cottonmouths, and copperheads.

Clinical features – These include anxiety with autonomic features, like nausea, vomiting, diaphoresis, diarrhea, and tachycardia. Local signs of envenomation are edema, erythema, ecchymoses, lymph node sweeping, oozing or weeping of the wound, and formation of bullae.

Systemic features of envenomation are diarrhea, confusion, vomiting, dyspnea hypotension, shock, and paresthesia. In rattlesnake bites, patients may complain of a metallic taste in their mouth. Envenomation by pit vipers can cause neuromuscular symptoms, like muscle weakness and muscle fasciculations. Patients can also present with anaphylaxis and coagulopathy.

Chapter 6: EMS Operations

This makes up 10% to 14% of test content. Topic areas include:

Ethical and Legal Issues

Ethical dilemmas

These are clinical scenarios and situations that involve the ethics of clinical practice. The principles of ethics in clinical practice include:

Fidelity – In clinical practice, the ethical principle of fidelity means that health workers are expected to keep all health information about their patients private and confidential. This ethical principle is breached when health workers discuss information about their patients with third parties. Something as simple as discussing the health conditions of patients with spouses who are not involved is a breach of fidelity.

Veracity – In ethical practice, health workers are expected to give their patients all the required truthful information needed to make informed consent.

Autonomy – This means patients have the final say in the way they receive treatment. The principle of autonomy works with informed consent. Patients must be educated on their condition and the indications of the treatment provided, including the side effects and complications. After this information is given, patients can then determine if they wish to receive treatment.

Beneficence – Health workers are expected to act in the best interest of patients.

Nonmaleficence – Health workers are expected not to harm patients, either intentionally or unintentionally. This principle addresses the issues of negligence, malpractice, and other breaches of civil law in medicolegal practice.

Justice – Health workers are required to be fair, impartial, and unbiased in the treatment of all patients regardless of their race, religion, tribe, sexual orientation, and sex.

Advance directives

In advance care planning, patients are allowed to make decisions about their health care management plans in case of crises. These decisions are often based on patients' values and discussions with loved ones and caregivers.

The principles of advance care planning include education on life-sustaining treatments available, making decisions on the forms of preferential treatment in the event of a life-limiting illness, discussing such plans with loved ones and caregivers, and filling out advance directives forms.

An advance directive is a written statement of a patient's preferential medical treatment at the end of life. It includes the living will, which is a legal document that states the forms of treatment patients prefer be administered if they are no longer able to give consent. These treatment options include resuscitation and other end-of-life treatment.

A health-care proxy or durable power of attorney is a document that states a patient's appointed attorney in cases when the person is unable to give consent. A durable power of attorney does not nullify the living will. Medical orders for life-sustaining treatment (MOLST) or Provider Orders for Life-Sustaining Treatment (POLST) are documents that contain the patient's medical orders for end-of-life treatment.

How to Lift and Move Patients

Principles of lifting patients

1. Before you lift a patient, assess the patient's weight and determine whether you need assistance in lifting.
2. To lift, use your legs to propel the patient upward. Do not use your waist.
3. Your feet should be planted squarely. Do not twist while lifting the patient.
4. Make sure the weight is close to your body.
5. Communicate clearly to your patient to reassure them.

How to lift stretchers and cots

1. It is advisable to use a stretcher with a mechanical lift.
2. Use a stair chair if it is available.
3. Assess the weight of the equipment and assess the number of hands you need. At least two people should be available to lift the equipment.
4. Before using the equipment to lift a patient, check the maximum amount of weight permitted for use.
5. Use the power lift or squat lift technique. These postures keep your back aligned and prevent straining of your pelvic muscles. The power lift is helpful for professionals with weak thighs or knees. To maintain this posture, keep your feet slightly apart. Your back should be straight, and the muscles in your anterior abdominal wall must be pushed in.
6. Your feet should be flat, and weight should be distributed equally to the balls of your feet.

7. To grip the object, bend your fingers at the same angles.
8. When lifting, do not bend at your waist.

How to carry equipment

1. It is safe to move objects on devices with wheels.
2. Before lifting, evaluate the weight of the equipment to be lifted.
3. Your back should be locked. Do not bend or twist your waist.
4. Avoid hyperextension of your back.
5. Work with other members of the team in an organized manner to prevent injury.
6. To carry equipment with one hand, keep your back straight. Do not lean to the other side to counterbalance the weight.
7. To carry equipment down the stairs, use a stair chair if available.
8. Your back should be locked and straight.
9. To reach for overhead equipment, lean from your hips and use the muscles in your shoulder to roll.
10. As much as possible, push the equipment rather than pull.
11. When pushing, your back should be locked and the weight close to the body.
12. Do not pull or push overhead weight.
13. Kneel to push/pull weight that is below your waist.
14. Your elbows should be bent and kept close to your sides.

Guidelines for moving patients

Indications for moving patients include fire or risk of fire; immediate danger; hazardous materials; the patient blocking access to patients in life-threatening conditions; inability to give care to patients in certain body postures or locations; and inability to protect patients from environmental hazards. Generally, patients with the following conditions should be moved: shock, altered consciousness, and ineffective breathing.

The greatest risk in moving trauma patients is the risk of worsening an existing spinal injury. To prevent this from happening, the patient should be pulled in the direction of the long axis of the spine. It is difficult to quickly extract a patient from a vehicle and simultaneously provide adequate protection to the cervical spine. You can move patients who are on the floor by dragging them on a blanket, tugging the shoulder and neck area of the patient's clothes, and grasping the forearms and pulling.

To extricate a patient caught under or in a vehicle, align their cervical spine into a neutral position by supporting the patient from behind and manually immobilizing the neck.

A second EMT puts the cervical collar in the patient, while a third person puts the backboard close to the door. The second person should support the patient's thorax while the third person extracts the legs from the pedal. At the prompting of the second person, both the first and third person should rotate the patient so that their back is in the door of the vehicle and their feet are propped on the passenger seat.

A bystander or another person should support the patient's head as the first person steps out to the vehicle, then resumes support of the patient's head.

The backboard is placed on top of the seat close to the patient's buttocks, and the patient is lowered on it. The other end of the backboard should be supported by assistants.

How to perform nonemergent moves

Direct ground lift without injury to the spine

1. Two to three rescuers should be on one side of the patient. They should be lined up.
2. The rescuers should kneel on one knee.
3. With the patient's arm on their own chest, Rescuer 1 should support the patient's neck with their arm and use their other arm to support the patient's back.
4. Rescuer 2 supports the patient's knees with one arm and the patient's buttocks with the other arm.
5. Rescuer 3 supports the patient's waist with both arms.
6. On cue, the patient is lifted to the rescuers' knees, then rolled toward their chests.
7. The patient is moved to the stretcher.

Extremity lift (with no injuries to the extremities)

1. Rescuer 1 kneels by the patient's head, and Rescuer 2 kneels by the patient's knees.
2. Rescuer 1 supports each of the patient's shoulders with their hands while Rescuer 2 holds the patient's wrists.
3. Rescuer 1 holds the patient's wrists by slipping their hands underneath the patient's arm; Rescuer 2 slips both hands underneath the patient's knees.
4. Rescuers 1 and 2 move to a crouching position in tandem.
5. Next, they stand up in tandem and transfer the patient to the stretcher.

How to transfer a supine patient from the bed to the stretcher

1. The cot should be placed perpendicular to the bed so that the head of the cot is to the door of the bed.
2. Unstrap the bed.

3. Two rescuers should stand between the stretcher and the bed, then face the patient.
4. Rescuer 1 slides their arm just underneath the patient's neck and holds the patient's shoulders.
5. Rescuer 2 slides a hand under the patient's hip and lifts it a bit.
6. Rescuer 1 slides their other arm under the patient's back while Rescuer 2 slides their arms under the patient's calves and hips.
7. Together, they slide the patient to the edge of the bed. The patient is then rotated and placed gently on the cot.

How to use the draw sheet method

1. Place the cot close to the bed and loosen the end of the bedsheet.
2. Unstrap the lower rails and adjust the cot height.
3. Grasp the ends of the sheet at the patient's head, chest, knees, and hips.
4. Slide the patient onto the cot.

How to position patients during transport

1. Patients with suspected injuries to the spine should be put in the recovery position.
2. Patients who complain of chest pain or breathlessness should be placed in the cardiac position as long as they are not hypotensive.
3. Immobilize all patients with suspected spinal injuries on a backboard.
4. Patients with hypoperfusion from hypovolemic shock should have their lower limbs elevated.
5. Pregnant patients with hypotension should be placed in the left lateral position.
6. Patients with nausea and vomiting should be placed in the lateral position to prevent choking on vomit.

Ambulance Operations

Steps for answering an ambulance call

1. **Preassignment and check**

This stage involves all the preparations and routine checks done before a distress call is received. Medical equipment is gathered and stored. Some of these tools include:

- Suction equipment
- Airway devices
- Oxygen units
- Oxygen delivery systems
- Artificial ventilation equipment
- Equipment for cardiac compression
- Supplies for wound care
- Supplies for splinting
- Supplies for childbirth
- Automated external defibrillator
- Medication
- Nonmedical equipment, like personal protective equipment
- Street maps and pre-planned routes

Apart from this, at this stage, the ambulance should be inspected for the following:

A. Fill the fuel tank and test the oil gauge, battery, brakes, and cooling system.
B. Inspect the ambulance tires and wheels for wear and tear.
C. Test the headlights, turn signals, emergency warning lights, siren, and horn.
D. Make sure that the air conditioning and communication system are functional.
E. Assess medical equipment for functionality (for example, check the defibrillator batteries and suction batteries). Spare batteries should always be available.

2. **Assignment operations**

At this stage, the call is received in the dispatch center by trained EMD personnel. The dispatcher asks the caller to provide information, like the nature of the call, the location of the patient, the name and location of the caller, the nature and severity of the patient's condition, and the number of patients.

En route to the location, seat belts should be worn at all times. Dispatch should be notified and essential information confirmed. Ambulance operators are expected to be mentally and physically fit, have a positive attitude, be tolerant, and be able to work under pressure. Drivers are expected to use the siren and red lights tactically. They should also use the proper route, keep a safe distance when driving, and follow all road safety guidelines.

Upon arrival at the scene, park the ambulance uphill from any liquid and leaking hazards and about 100 feet away from the scene. Red lights should be turned off, and warning lights should be used. Do not park in a place that can block an exit. All local and state laws concerning the use of emergency vehicles and ambulance escorts should be followed. These laws affect the parking of ambulances, speed limits, routes for emergency response, use of stop signs and red lights, and use of visual and auditory alert systems.

For safety, multiple vehicle responses should be used only if the location of the patient or facility is unfamiliar. Multiple vehicle responses can cause crashes at intersections and collide with other motorists.

3. At the scene

At this stage, the dispatcher should be notified that the ambulance has arrived. Next, assess the situation for hazards and perform the body isolation protocol. During the assessment, note the type of injury (medical or surgical incident). Determine the number of affected patients. Commence triage promptly, and stabilize the cervical spine if necessary. Call for extra help if necessary.

At the scene, quickly provide emergency care. Prep the patient for transport and transfer to the vehicle. Assess dressings, slings, and all critical care interventions. On the way to the facility, notify the dispatch technician and complete and record all ongoing assessments.

Notify the receiving facility and complete all reports. At the facility, notify the dispatch technician. Transfer the patient and complete all reports. On the way back to the station, notify the dispatch technician. Prepare for the next call. Clean the ambulance, refuel, and file all reports.

4. Accessing and extracting the patient

In nonrescue emergency cases, EMTs are expected to provide care to patients before extraction and ensure that patients are extracted from the hazardous environment. Nonrescue EMS professionals must collaborate with rescuers in such a way that they do not let their activities interfere with the emergency care provided to patients. A chain of command should be followed to ensure that care is provided. Patient care is prioritized above extraction unless extraction can put the patient at risk of death.

Safety guidelines

1. Use the appropriate protective equipment.
2. To ensure the patient's safety, inform and obtain consent from all conscious patients before extraction.
3. Protect the patient from sharp metal, broken glass, and other hazards.
4. To access the patient, try opening the doors and rolling down the windows. If possible, ask the patient to unlock the doors. Sometimes access can be possible only through the use of special equipment and tools.
5. Before extracting the patient, stabilize and immobilize the cervical spine.

Incident Management

The national incident management system is made up of principles, concepts, and doctrines that regulate how incidents are responded to. The components include command and management, resource management, communications and information management, preparedness, ongoing management, and supporting technologies.

Command and management – Responses to all forms of hazards are standardized across government levels based on the use of public information systems, multiagency coordination systems, and incident command systems.

Preparedness – This component is responsible for measuring and establishing the abilities of agencies.

Resource management – This standardizes the way inventory is tracked and described before, during, and after the management of an incident.

Communications and information management – This component manages communication and information shared during an incident.

Supporting technologies – This provides technology and systems that support the management of critical incidents.

Types of disasters

Natural disasters – Hurricanes, winter storms, tornados, and floods

Technical hazards – Hazmat incidents, the collapse of buildings

Transportation accidents – Affecting rail, road, ship, and aircraft

Civil unrest – Strikes, demonstrations, and riots

Terrorist and criminal incidents

Mass casualty incidents
These are incidents with injuries affecting a large number of people and can overwhelm available resources in a region.

Goals of management

1. Use resources judiciously.
2. Provide care to a large number of people.
3. Do not relocate the incident.
4. Prioritize patients.

Initial response to mass casualties
Initial response – On arrival, EMS professionals should triage each patient to prioritize care. Resist the initial response to provide detailed one-on-one care to each victim. Also, for the sake of organization and coordination, the first EMS team to appear at the scene is in charge.

Assess the safety of the environment – Assess for likely hazards that can make the environment unsafe for both patients and responders (such as fire, nuclear agents, biologic agents, electrical hazards, flammable liquids, secondary explosions, debris, and more).

Assess incident scene – Also assess the scene of the incident for the extent of damage, number of injured people, number of patients with severe injuries, and more.

Report – Report the situation to a dispatcher to send backup. Also report the situation to the medical command center.

Set up – Organize the scene for management of casualties. To do this, triage each patient and secure the space for work.

Triage
Triage makes it possible for responders and EMS professionals to quickly assess and assign all victims into groups. It also makes it possible for professionals to quickly assign and provide emergency care and transport patients to receiving centers. Because patients are prioritized according to urgency of care and transportation, all patients are attended to and available resources are used judiciously. Furthermore, triaging patients with minor injuries reduces workload and inflow of patients into the receiving center.

The START model of triage

START means Simple Triage And Rapid Treatment. This model assesses and categorizes patients based on mental status, circulation, and respiration.

1. Start from where you are and begin assessing patients.
2. Categorize patients into green, yellow, red, and black tags.
3. Begin by locating patients who can stand and walk. Make an announcement encouraging patients who can stand to do so.
4. Tag those patients with a green ribbon. These patients should be relocated.
5. Move in an organized fashion, assessing patients' breathing, circulation, and mental status.
6. Tag patients accordingly with a ribbon.
7. Keep tabs on the number of patients.
8. Secondary triaging can be done in the treatment area, on the stretcher, or in an ambulance en route to the receiving center.

Red tag (immediate) – Patients in this category require immediate treatment.

Yellow (delayed) – Patients in this category can have treatment delayed for a few minutes until patients in the red tags are stabilized.

Green (minor) – Patients in this category are stable with minor injuries to soft tissues and/or swollen deformities of bones and joints.

Black (dead/cannot be helped) – Patients in this category have the least priority. These patients are either clinically dead or in a state where resuscitation is of no benefit.

Response to Terrorism and Hazmat

Incident size-up – This includes assessment of the type of material, confirmation of the type of hazmat, the extent of contamination, and more. EMS professionals should be highly suspicious of incidents affecting transportation, manufacturing plants, terrorism, crashes on highways, tankers, tractors, railroads, mass storage facilities, pipelines, warehouses, chemical plants, shopping centers, laboratories, health-care centers, agricultural facilities, and others.

Identifying hazards
Vehicles should be labeled with hazards. Some common UN/DOT placards include gases, explosives, flammable solids, flammable liquids, organic peroxides and oxidizers, corrosives, radioactive material, and miscellaneous.

Red labels signify fire hazards. Yellow labels signify radioactive hazards. Blue labels signify health hazards.

Zones of hazardous materials

Hot zone – This zone is the area of contamination (the site of the release of hazardous materials). High-level PPE must be used to enter this zone. Also, the entry must be restricted to professionals skilled in working with hazmat incidents.

Warm zone – This is a buffer area just outside the hot zone. It is located close to the decontamination corridor. Access to this area is restricted to trained professionals.

Cold zone – This area is safe, and EMS professionals can monitor and attend to patients here. This area is used to stage equipment and personnel.

Types of contamination
Primary contamination – The contaminants come in direct contact with the patient.

Secondary contamination – A contaminated person comes in contact with equipment and/or personnel.

Substances with the highest risks for secondary contamination include very toxic solids and liquids, like organophosphates; biological agents, like viruses and bacteria; and radioactive dust and liquids. These substances easily cling to the skin, hair, and clothing of contaminated victims. Substances with little risk for contamination include carbon monoxide, motor oil, amine gases, propylene glycol, and others.

Absorption of poisons
Topical route – Via the skin and mucous membranes. Not all poisons are absorbed at the same rate.

Inhalation route – Poisons are absorbed via the mucosa in the respiratory airway.

Gastrointestinal route – Poisons are absorbed via the oral cavity.

Parenteral route – Poisons are absorbed via wounds, injections, and invasive procedures.

How to decontaminate

Dilution – Lavage with large amounts of normal saline or water. Dilution decreases the concentration of the poison and reduces the rate of absorption.

Absorption – Pads and towels are used to mop up the material. It is used after lavage and for environmental poisons.

Neutralization – This is a rare form of decontamination due to the risk of exothermic reaction and time needed to determine the exact neutralizing material.

Disposal/isolation – The patient is quickly removed from the source of exposure. Also, all clothing is removed and the patient is exposed.

Levels of PPE

Level A protection – This is the highest form of PPE. It includes an encapsulated suit and a self-contained breathing apparatus. The suit is sealed and impermeable to chemicals, aerosols, and other hazmat incidents. It is used to access the hot zone of contamination.

Level B protection – This is nonencapsulating, with the self-containing breathing apparatus worn outside the suit. However, it is easier to use. It is used by the decontamination team.

Level C protection – This suit is worn to move contaminated patients. It protects personnel from secondary contamination. The clothing is nonpermeable.

Level D protection – An example of this is the uniform used by firefighters.

Terrorism

Infrastructures that are prone to terrorist attacks include school and recreational facilities, mass transit, economic centers, telecommunications centers, water supplies, electrical grids, medical facilities, research facilities, and places of cultural and historical significance, etc.

Classification of weapons of mass destruction

Chemical agents

Choking agents – Diphosgene, phosgene, chloropicrin, and chlorine. These chemicals irritate the mucosa in the respiratory tree, oral cavity, and eyes. They cause pulmonary edema and secondary pneumonia.

Blister agents – Sulfur mustard arsenicals, nitrogen mustard, and phosgene oxime. These chemicals irritate the eyes and skin and, when inhaled, irritate the respiratory mucosa.

Blood agents – Cyanogen chloride and hydrogen cyanide. These chemicals affect the central nervous system. They block oxygenation of the red blood cells and prevent cells from using oxygen.

Nerve agents – Soman, sarin, tabun, and V-agent. Cholinesterases prevent the breakdown of acetylcholine. These chemicals stimulate the acetylcholine receptors and cause parasympathetic hyperactivity. Symptoms include lacrimation, diarrhea, fasciculations, miosis, salivation, urinary incontinence, vomiting, and convulsions.

Biological agents

These include infectious viruses, bacteria, and biological toxins extracted from plants, animals, and microbes. Examples include bacteria (plague, anthrax, and Q fever), viruses (Ebola and smallpox), toxins (ricin, botulinum, and enterotoxin B from staphylococcus aureus).

Radiologic agents

Radiologic agents contain particles that affect cells. These particles include alpha, gamma, and beta particles. These are absorbed by the body and cause acute and chronic cellular inflammation.

Indicators of use of weapons of mass destruction

Primary indicators include mass casualties, similar symptoms among victims, the discovery of dissemination devices, evidence from detectors, warnings, and/or credit taken by terrorists.

Secondary indicators include mass death of birds and animals, laboratory test reports, and statements from victims.

Dissemination devices

Direct deposit – This is a mechanical device that can be controlled easily with no collateral damage. Agents can be fitted into pens, cans, and umbrellas.

Breaking devices – These are mechanical devices with a point source. They cover the agent, which is released when the device is broken.

Bursting/exploding devices – These devices disseminate the agent through an explosion.

Spraying devices – These are mechanical devices that encapsulate an agent reservoir. They use pressure to spread the agent.

Vectors – These are biologic carriers of biologic agents (insects, small mammals, food, and fomites).

Test 1: Questions

1. You are called to see a 65-year-old hypertensive female with squeezing chest pain that radiates down her left arm to her neck and jaw. She says her heartbeat is faster, she is having difficulty breathing, and she has felt weak for the past couple of days. Which of the following is the most appropriate first step for this patient?

   A. Secure IV access.
   B. Place her in a comfortable position and administer supplemental oxygen.
   C. Do an ECG and defibrillate if there is an irregular rhythm.
   D. Carry out an initial assessment looking for any immediate threats to life.

2. Your team gets a call from an elderly female in the summer. Her 83-year-old husband, who has been vomiting and passing frequent loose stools for the past week, has passed out. You get there and find the man lying supine on the floor with shallow breathing and RR of 32 cpm. His lips are dry; his skin is cold; and his pulse is 128 beats per minute, weak, and thready. His BP is 78/50 mmHg. What is the cause of this presentation?

   A. Septic shock
   B. Psychogenic shock
   C. Anaphylactic shock
   D. Dehydration

3. You are carrying out a preliminary assessment on a 27-year-old female who was run over by a drunk driver while crossing the street. She is lying supine in a pool of blood and is lethargic, with agonal breathing and multiple abrasions, lacerations, and a crush injury on her left leg. Her skin is also cold and clammy because of shunting of blood to vital organs. Which organ is most important?

   A. The heart
   B. The brain
   C. The lungs
   D. The kidneys

4. A 22-year-old pregnant female in her first trimester starts bleeding profusely from her vagina after spotting for the past two days. On your arrival at her home, she is conscious, cold but weak, with a heart rate of 132 bpm, respiratory rate of 28 cpm, and BP of 92/60 mmHg. Which of the following actions is most appropriate?

   A. Placing her in a supine position and administering supplemental oxygen
   B. Securing IV access and starting an infusion to increase blood volume
   C. Placing her in the modified Trendelenburg position
   D. Starting her on supplemental oxygen

5. You are called by neighbors to attend to a middle-aged diabetic man who was robbed at home and pushed down a flight of stairs by his assailant. You find him lying at the foot of the stairs, conscious but complaining of a headache where he hit his head. His skin is warm, and his breathing is labored with a pulse rate of 40 cpm and a BP of 80/48 mmHg. The man has no visible injuries. What is the most likely cause of his presentation?

A. Hypovolemia
B. Trauma to his cervical spine
C. Hypoglycemic shock
D. Myocardial ischemia

6. Your team is called to the scene of an accident where a sports car ran into an electric pole at high speed. The sole driver of the vehicle has managed to stumble out but has a shard of glass through his right arm, which is not actively bleeding. You determine scene safety; establish there is one patient; and, on primary assessment, discover that he is conscious but disoriented with a good pulse, respiration, and blood pressure. Which of the following will the patient most benefit from?

A. Pull out the shard of glass, then apply direct pressure to the wound.
B. Elevate the arm above the patient's head, then pull out the shard of glass.
C. Apply a tourniquet proximal to the injury, then pull out the shard of glass.
D. Apply a tourniquet proximal to the injury and leave the shard in.

7. You want to apply a tourniquet on a 48-year-old male who slit his left wrist in a suicide attempt. Which of the following steps is not part of the procedure?

A. Wrapping your bandage distal to the slit
B. Using a stick as a handle to secure the bandage
C. Writing "TK" on the patient's forehead
D. Folding a triangular bandage into four in a cravat

8. A 51-year-old female complains of burning chest pain radiating to her back, palpitations, and dizziness. She was diagnosed with hypertension 12 years ago but has been unable to take her medications in the last month. Her BP is 138/100 mmHg; her pulse rate is 30 cpm, and she is having difficulty breathing. Which of the following actions is most appropriate?

A. Place the patient in a comfortable position, administer oxygen, and transport her quickly to a hospital.
B. Allow the patient to rest in a comfortable position and administer nitroglycerin, as it is most likely angina.
C. Give the patient antacids to relieve her peptic ulcer symptoms.
D. Take a detailed history from the patient and her family.

9. You are called to an office complex where a 65-year-old male suddenly felt lightheaded with severe chest pain, which he describes as stabbing in nature. In your preliminary assessment, you discover that the man's blood pressure is 89/60 mmHg with a weak radial pulse of 118 bpm and a respiratory rate of 38 cpm. Your colleague, who is assisting, counts a pulse of 96 bpm in the man's other wrist. What is the most likely cause of this presentation?

A. Aortic dissection
B. Angina
C. Neurogenic shock
D. Congestive cardiac failure

10. Your team is called to attend to a university professor who suddenly felt faint during a presentation. Her husband tells you she was diagnosed with hypertension 33 years ago but takes antihypertensives only when her blood pressure is elevated. The woman complains of breathlessness and is coughing up pinkish sputum. On assessment, you find that she has a respiratory rate of 26 cpm and SaO2 of 94% with a wheeze and crackles on auscultation. Her BP is 70/62 mmHg with cold extremities. What is the most likely cause of this presentation?

A. Neurogenic shock
B. Asthma exacerbation
C. Cardiogenic shock
D. Anaphylactic shock

11. In an emergency you are giving CPR to a patient as the sole EMT. Which of the following is accurate about the methodology?

A. 30 chest compressions followed by 20 rescue breaths
B. 2 chest compressions followed by 30 rescue breaths
C. 30 chest compressions followed by 3 rescue breaths
D. 30 chest compressions followed by 2 rescue breaths

12. In an emergency, you are using an automated external defibrillator on a patient. Which of the following is correct about the methodology?

A. CPR and defibrillation should be done simultaneously.
B. One shock should be followed by immediate CPR, beginning with rescue breaths.
C. Analyze the patient's rhythm after five minutes of CPR.
D. Chest compressions and artificial ventilation should be stopped when shocks are being delivered.

13. Your team is transporting a 56-year-old patient with suspected myocardial infarction to the hospital when suddenly he loses consciousness, he stops breathing, and his pulse is no longer palpable. Which of the following should not be part of your treatment regimen?

A. Rush the patient to the hospital while your coresponders administer CPR.
B. Stop the vehicle, commence CPR, and use the AED once it is ready.
C. Analyze rhythm and deliver one shock if prompted by the AED.
D. If a "no shock" message is delivered and no pulse is present, resume CPR and continue transport to the hospital.

14. In delivering high-quality CPR, which of the following is not correct according to AHA guidelines?

A. Chest compressions should be hard, fast, and at least 2 inches/5 centimeters in depth.
B. Allow as much ventilation as possible.
C. Allow complete chest recoil.
D. Change compressor every two minutes or sooner if fatigued.

15. Which of the following is not part of an emergency medical responder's job in an emergency scenario?

A. Verify scene safety.
B. Activate the emergency response system via a mobile device.
C. Assess for breathing and pulse simultaneously within 10 seconds.
D. If breathing is not present but pulse is felt, start CPR with cycles of 30 chest compressions and three breaths.

16. You are called to a bank where a 35-year-old male has suddenly slumped over. He has agonal breathing with a weak, thready pulse. Bystanders say the man clutched his chest before collapsing. Which of the following steps is most appropriate?

A. Monitor the man's vitals until the AED arrives.
B. Provide chest compressions until the AED arrives.
C. Provide rescue breathing of 10 breaths/min; check pulse every two minutes and commence CPR if it is absent.
D. Provide rescue breathing of 15 breaths/min; check pulse every two minutes and commence CPR if it is absent.

17. Upon arriving at the scene of an armed robbery, you find a security guard who fell after being pistol-whipped, hitting his head against the tiled floor. There is a pool of blood around his head and dark circles around both eyes. He is unconscious with a respiratory rate of 30 cpm and a pulse rate of 120 bpm . He has cold limbs. To administer high-concentration oxygen effectively, which of the following is applicable?

A. Do a head-tilt/chin-lift maneuver to open the airway.
B. Use a nasopharyngeal airway to ensure the airway is patent.
C. Use cricoid pressure to ensure airway patency.
D. Do a jaw thrust without head extension to open the airway.

18. You are attending to a 27-year-old gymnast who complains of tearing substernal chest pain of one day's duration, which intensified while he was training at the gym. He confesses he has been taking self-prescribed amitriptyline for his clinical depression and has not been to see his doctor in over six months. While you are talking to the man, he suddenly looks panicked and slumps. He has no pulse, he has no recordable blood pressure, and no respiratory effort is noticeable. What is your next course of action?

A. Apply the AED and start defibrillation immediately.
B. Start chest compressions immediately, giving 30 chest compressions followed by two breaths while waiting for an AED.
C. Start rescue breathing, giving one breath every six seconds while waiting for an AED.
D. Move the patient to the vehicle for immediate transportation.

19. A 22-year-old female wakes up with difficulty breathing, excruciating chest pain, and a cough producing yellowish sputum. She also has severe right shoulder pain, which began suddenly while driving home from work yesterday. She is pale and warm to the touch. Her respiratory rate is 34 cpm. SpO2 is 90% with a pulse rate of 100 bpm. The woman volunteers that her genotype is SS. Which of the following interventions is most appropriate?

A. Commence supplementary oxygen and keep the patient warm.
B. Move the patient to the vehicle for immediate transportation to the hospital.
C. Support the patient's respiration with a BVM and oxygen.
D. Call 911 and follow the instructions.

20. A 51-year-old female who thinks she was bitten on her right foot by a snake a few hours ago while gardening says she has been continuously bleeding from the bite site and noticed blood on her gums. Which of the following will be least beneficial for this patient?

A. Ensure scene safety for yourself and the patient.
B. Apply a tourniquet proximal to the bite site.
C. Reassure the patient she will not die from the snakebite.
D. Ensure airway, breathing, and circulation, and give oxygen if appropriate.

21. The functions of the respiratory system include all except which of the following?

A. Filtration of particulate matter from circulation
B. Water balance
C. Metabolism of certain drugs and enzymes
D. Tissue respiration by uptake of CO_2

22. At the scene of an automobile accident, the patient is lying unconscious. Which of the following maneuvers is required in opening up the airway if neck injury is suspected?

A. Head-tilt/chin-lift
B. Jaw thrust
C. Modified head-thrust
D. Neck-tilt

23. A 55-year-old obese female complains of sudden onset of breathlessness, unilateral left leg swelling, lower calf pain, and chest pain after a 12-hour flight. You auscultate and hear a localized wheeze. Blood pressure is 150/90 mmHg. Pulse rate is 114 bpm; oxygen saturation is SaO_2 80%. What is the appropriate intervention?

A. Administer a corticosteroid inhaler.
B. Elevate the foot of the bed.
C. Commence chest compressions.
D. Administer oxygen.

24. Parts of the upper airway include all except which of the following?

A. Mouth
B. Nostril
C. Nasopharynx
D. Trachea

25. Choose the best answer option concerning inspiration.
   A. The chest cavity decreases in size.
   B. The diaphragm moves downward and inward.
   C. The diaphragm relaxes, and the ribs are moved outward by the intercostal muscles.
   D. Inspiration produces a slight negative pressure inside the thoracic cavity.

26. Which of the following is a part of the lower airway?
   A. Larynx
   B. Pharynx
   C. Nares
   D. Bronchioles

27. What is the primary drive for respiratory control?
   A. Reduced oxygen saturation in the blood
   B. Increased carbon dioxide saturation in the blood
   C. Reduced lung compliance
   D. Reduced hemoglobin concentration in blood

28. A 70-year-old COPD patient complains of shortness of breath. He is dyspneic, cyanosed, flaring, and breathing with accessory muscles. He can barely complete a sentence. His respiratory rate is 30 cpm; SaO2 is 90%. On auscultation, crackles are heard in the lower lung zones with diminished breath sounds. Which of the following is the most likely reason for the man's distress?
   A. Respiratory distress
   B. Respiratory failure
   C. Respiratory arrest
   D. Cardiac arrest

29. A 30-year-old female is visibly shaken and hysterical after a robbery. Her respiratory rate is 28 breaths/minute, blood pressure 160/90 mmHg, pulse rate 116 bpm , and SPO2 95%. What should you do?
   A. Administer oxygen via a nasal cannula.
   B. Reassure the patient and perform a secondary assessment.
   C. Encourage the patient to breathe into a paper bag.
   D. Administer an antihypertensive.

30. A 60-year-old female with a history of COPD is having difficulty remaining alert. She looks tired. Her skin is cool and clammy. Blood pressure is 140/90, pulse 120 bpm, SaO2 90%, respiration 10 cpm. Which of the following steps is appropriate?

A. Commence BVM ventilation.
B. Give oxygen via a non-rebreather mask.
C. Commence CPR.
D. Assist the patient with a prescribed corticosteroid inhaler.

31. A 28-year-old female with a history of allergic dermatitis and rhinitis presents with sudden onset dyspnea, chest tightness, and wheezing after exposure to pollen dust. She admits to occasional nonproductive night coughs before the incident. She is afebrile. Her blood pressure is 100/6 0mmHg, pulse rate 84 bpm, respiratory rate is 26 breaths per minute. SaO2 is 94%, and rhonchi are heard on auscultation. What is the most likely prehospital diagnosis for this patient?

A. Bronchiolitis
B. Bronchiectasis
C. Asthma
D. Cystic fibrosis

32. The pathophysiology of the above patient's condition is caused by which of the following?

A. Airway inflammation
B. Airway hyperresponsiveness
C. Airflow limitation
D. All of the above

33. A 16-year-old male is receiving artificial ventilation after a near-drowning incident. He is peripherally cyanosed and apneic. His pulse rate is 40 bpm, weak, and low in volume. His blood pressure is 80/50 mmHg, and his breath sounds are diminished in lung zones. As an EMT attending to this patient, how will you know he is being adequately ventilated?

A. Chest rises and falls with each ventilation.
B. Heart rate decreases.
C. Persistent cyanosis.
D. None of the above.

34. While resuscitating an unconscious patient, copious secretions cover the oropharynx. You use a mobile suction machine on the patient. What amount of vacuum pressure should a properly functioning suction unit generate?

A. 250 mmHg
B. 200 mmHg
C. 300 mmHg
D. 400 mmHg

35. A 50-year-old male with a medical history of chronic bronchitis, type 2 diabetes, and hypertension is in acute respiratory failure. He is drowsy, lethargic, and responsive to painful stimuli. As an EMT at the scene, which of the following airway adjuncts should you use while providing positive pressure ventilation for this patient?

A. Nasopharyngeal airway
B. Laryngeal mask airway
C. Laryngoscope
D. Non-rebreather mask

36. A 29-year-old male presents unconscious at home after an evening out with his friends. He has multiple needle marks on his left forearm, is unresponsive, and is making loud snoring sounds. His breathing rate is 8 breaths per minute and shallow. His pulse is 60 bpm, and his blood pressure is 90/60 mmHg. What intervention should you take?

A. Commence cardiopulmonary resuscitation.
B. Give oxygen using a non-rebreather mask.
C. Insert an oropharyngeal airway and begin ventilation.
D. Lay the patient in the left recumbent position.

37. A 72-year-old female who has a medical history of COPD, bronchial asthma, and a significant history of smoking complains of sudden onset dyspnea and left-sided chest pain after lifting a heavy weight. She is in respiratory distress and speaking in short sentences. Her respiratory rate is 28 breaths per minute; pulse rate is 114 bpm, blood pressure 130/60 mmHg, and SaO2 is 92% on room air. The woman has a rescue inhaler she uses occasionally. On auscultation, breath sounds are absent in the left upper lung zones with hyperresonant percussion notes. What intervention should you take?

A. Help the patient into a comfortable position and administer supplemental oxygen.
B. Give the patient her prescribed rescue inhaler.
C. Encourage the patient to breathe into a paper bag.
D. Give oral acetaminophen for chest pain.

38. A 70-year-old male with a significant history of smoking and alcohol intake complains of chronic cough with minimal expectoration of five years duration. He is dyspneic at rest, has pursed-lip breathing, and is rail-thin and flushed in appearance. Audible wheezing can be heard. He has a prescribed rescue inhaler. Pulse is 104 bpm, and SaO2 is 85% on room air. What is the most likely prehospital diagnosis?

A. Chronic bronchitis
B. Bronchial asthma
C. Emphysema
D. None of the above

39. Which of the following most accurately describes the pathophysiology of emphysema?

A. Destruction of lung parenchyma, leading to loss of elastic recoil and alveolar destruction
B. Collapse of lung tissue with loss of volume
C. Hypersensitive airway responsiveness
D. Viral lung infection and subsequent inflammation

40. Patients with emphysema are called pink puffers for which of the following reasons?

A. Polycythemia from hypoxia
B. Increased epinephrine production
C. Hyperventilation
D. Increased blood supply to the skin

41. A 60-year-old male with a medical history of COPD and coronary artery disease complains of sudden-onset dyspnea and shortness of breath. Shortness of breath has progressively worsened for four days since he had a sore throat, and he is unable to speak in full sentences. He has chest pain and coughs up purulent, yellow sputum. He also complains of bilateral leg swelling. On examination, he is febrile, stocky in appearance, and cyanosed, which worsens during coughing spells. He also has distended neck veins. Pulse rate is 96 bpm and regular. Respiratory rate is 30 breaths per minutes, and SaO2 is 86%. As the EMT at the scene, what should you do?

A. Determine the man's blood pressure.
B. Give high-flow oxygen via a non-rebreather mask.
C. Give supplemental oxygen using a Venturi mask.
D. Administer the prescribed rescue inhaler.

42. What percentage of oxygen does a Venturi mask deliver?

A. 96%–100%
B. 90%–96%
C. 20%–65%
D. 24%–60%

43. A 30-year-old female is sitting upright in bed; she is dyspneic and anxious. She speaks in short sentences and takes deep breaths. She wheezes while trying to breathe out. She also complains of a dry, nonproductive cough, which worsens in the evening. She has dry, eczematous skin that itches, and she has scratch marks all over her body. Which of the following is an appropriate intervention?

A. Avoid oral corticosteroids.
B. Administer injectable epinephrine.
C. Administer oxygen using a non-rebreather mask.
D. Give the patient inhaled bronchodilators using a metered-dose inhaler.

44. You are called to attend to a 34-year-old female in a restaurant who is having difficulty breathing and speaking in a muffled tone. Onlookers say she was having a peanut butter sandwich for lunch when she suddenly became breathless. On examination, the patient's skin is cool and pale, respiratory rate is 24 cpm, and wheezing can be heard bilaterally on auscultation of her lungs. Her blood pressure is 90/70 mmHG, with a heart rate of 100 bpm. What is the first step you should take in treating this patient?

A. Give the patient an epinephrine injection.
B. Administer high-flow oxygen via a non-rebreather.
C. Encourage the patient to cough continuously.
D. Perform an abdominal thrust.

45. A conscious 65-year-old male is noticed to be having difficulty breathing. On examination, he purses his lips as he tries to exhale, and he uses his accessory muscles of respiration. He appears thin, and his skin is pink. There is a history of cigarette smoking, and SaO2 is 92%. How will you manage this patient?

A. Ask him to sit up with his legs hanging off the bed.
B. Supply oxygen via BVM.
C. Administer low-flow oxygen via nasal cannula.
D. Collect a further history from the patient.

46. A 69-year-old female is found lying unresponsive with shallow respiration at a rate of 6 cpm. She has overdosed on her opioid analgesic medication. What is the next step in this patient's management?

A. Insert an oropharyngeal airway.
B. Stabilize the patient's cervical spine.
C. Administer low-dose oxygen via a nasal cannula.
D. Administer IV naltrexone.

47. During a practice session, a 16-year-old football player develops sudden onset of left-sided chest pain and breathlessness. On examination, his respiratory rate is 28 cpm, heart rate is 108 bpm, and blood pressure is 110/70 mmHg. His breath sounds are diminished on the left side of his chest, and his oxygen saturation is 94%. What should you do?

A. Help the patient into a comfortable position.
B. Administer the patient's prescribed inhaler.
C. Administer analgesics.
D. Commence BVM ventilation.

48. A 12-year-old female is in respiratory distress but is alert and responsive. She complains of feeling a tightness in her chest and struggles to complete sentences. You notice she uses accessory muscles for respiration and has an audible wheeze. What should you do next?

A. Assist the patient with her prescribed multidose inhaler.
B. Encourage the patient to breathe into a paper bag.
C. Commence BVM ventilation.
D. Encourage the patient to sit in a comfortable position.

49. You are attending to a 3-year-old female who was carried in by her parents. They tell you she has had a fever for the past three days and a cough that is raspy with a harsh sound heard on respiration. What is the most likely diagnosis?

A. Bronchopneumonia
B. Bronchiolitis
C. Croup
D. Common cold

50. You are the EMT responding to a call from a 54-year-old female with difficulty breathing. She reports feeling cold and experiencing flu-like symptoms in the last 12 days. There is chest pain when she coughs, with production of yellow sputum. Auscultation of the woman's lungs reveals crackles, and her oxygen saturation is 95%. What should be done for this patient?

A. Administer chest compressions.
B. Administer oxygen via BVM.
C. Assist the patient into a comfortable position.
D. Administer low-flow oxygen via a nasal cannula.

51. You are called to attend to a 53-year-old female with sudden onset chest pain. She has no history of trauma; however, she was on a long-distance flight the previous weekend. On auscultation, you hear a wheeze in the right lower side of her chest. There is also a positive smoking history. This is the first time the woman is having these symptoms. What is the most likely diagnosis?

A. Bronchopneumonia
B. Pulmonary embolism
C. COPD
D. Asthma

52. A 16-year-old male is preparing for a school quiz, which is scheduled to start in an hour. He suddenly becomes breathless and anxious. He also reports numbness around his face and hands. His blood pressure is 138/85 mmHg, with a heart rate of 100 bpm. He is breathing 30 times per minute. What should you do?

A. Encourage the patient to use a prescribed inhaler.
B. Administer oxygen to the patient via a nasal cannula.
C. Encourage the patient to breathe into a paper bag.
D. Collect further history from the patient.

53. You are called to attend to a 65-year-old male who complains of epigastric pain, which started suddenly while he was taking a walk. He also feels pain around his jaw, and he is diaphoretic. His blood pressure is 130/80 mmHg with a pulse of 98 bpm. What is the next step in managing this patient?

A. Take a further history.
B. Prescribe antiulcer medication.
C. Assist the patient in taking his prescribed nitroglycerin tablet.
D. Place the patient in the lateral recumbent position.

54. A 53-year-old male is found sitting by a sidewalk, breathless. He complains of weakness. You notice he has pedal edema. On auscultation, he has bilateral crackles in his lungs. His oxygen saturation is 94%, respiratory rate is 30 cpm, heart rate is 98 bpm, and blood pressure is 145/90 mmHg. Which of the following will improve this man's condition?

A. Administer oxygen via a nasal cannula.
B. Help the man sit properly and perform further assessment.
C. Administer an antihypertensive.
D. Encourage the man to lie in the supine position.

55. You are called to attend to a 45-year-old male who complains of sudden, tearing chest pain. On examination, you notice a respiratory rate of 30 cpm and a thready pulse rate of 110 bpm. Blood pressure is 90/60 mmHg. What is the most likely diagnosis?

A. Septic shock
B. Aortic dissection
C. Tension pneumothorax
D. Acute coronary syndrome

56. You are called to attend to a 16-year-old female who has been febrile the last week. She is lying in bed and complains of weakness, diarrhea, and vomiting. You notice her skin is pale and dry with areas of purpura. Oxygen saturation is 95%; her pulse and respiratory rates are elevated with a blood pressure of 100/60 mmHg. Which of the following interventions is appropriate?

A. Encourage the patient to sit upright in bed.
B. Administer supplemental oxygen.
C. Perform a secondary assessment.
D. Prescribe antidiarrheal medication.

57. Concerning CPR, which of the following is incorrect?

A. For adults, administer at least 100 compressions per minute.
B. Begin CPR with chest compressions before ventilation.
C. For adults, space ventilation so that three breaths are delivered after every 20 compressions.
D. For pediatric patients, compress the chest to a depth of at least one-third to one-half of the total depth.

58. You are called to see a 43-year-old male with peptic ulcer disease. He complains of nausea; weakness; and passage of loose stools, which are dark red to black. He was out with his friends last night and drank a lot of alcohol. His blood pressure is 100/70, with tachypnea and tachycardia. Which of the following is the most likely cause of this presentation?

A. Food poisoning
B. Dehydration
C. Anaphylaxis
D. Gastrointestinal bleeding

59. A 63-year-old patient experiences breathlessness and chest discomfort. While you are carrying out a preliminary examination, he suddenly collapses and becomes unresponsive. Which of the following is the correct sequence of management?

A. Apply AED pads, begin CPR, check for a carotid pulse.
B. Check for a carotid pulse, begin CPR, apply AED pads.
C. Begin CPR, check for a carotid pulse, apply AED pads.
D. Apply AED pads, check for a carotid pulse, begin CPR.

60. Concerning sickle cell disease, which of the following is false?

A. It is more common in African Americans and Africans.
B. It occurs due to sickling of defective red blood cells.
C. Sickled cells have a longer life span and more oxygen-carrying capacity.
D. If two sickle cell carriers have children, each child has one-fourth of a chance of developing the disease.

61. A 7-year-old child complains of chest pain and swelling of the hands and feet. You also notice a yellow tinge in his eyes. Both parents are carriers of the sickle cell trait. Which of the following is the patient most likely suffering from?

A. Vaso-occlusive crisis
B. Heart failure
C. Hemophilia
D. Dubin-Johnson syndrome

62. According to the Cincinnati prehospital stroke scale, which of the following is correct?

A. Facial droop – Patients can show their teeth.
B. Arm drift – Patients close their eyes and extend both hands straight out for five seconds.
C. Speech – Patients can say their name repeatedly.
D. Facial droop – Patients extend their tongue.

63. A 59-year-old male has had a stroke. He complains of headaches, nausea, and vomiting. On examination, you notice bilateral limb weakness and blurry vision. Which cerebral vessel is most likely affected?

A. Left internal carotid artery
B. Basilar artery
C. Right internal carotid artery
D. Middle cerebral artery

64. You are called to attend to a 15-year-old male who is having jerky arm movements. There is also involuntary micturition but no loss of consciousness. What kind of seizure is this?

A. Complex partial seizure
B. Absence seizure
C. Simple partial seizure
D. Myoclonic seizure

65. Which of the following is false about West syndrome?

A. It is a rare disorder in infancy and early childhood.
B. It is also called infantile spasm.
C. There is no mental retardation.
D. It includes congenital abnormalities, hydrocephalus, and epilepsy.

66. Concerning Lennox-Gastaut syndrome, which of the following is false?

A. It may cause developmental delays in children.
B. Sufferers of this condition have behavioral problems.
C. Seizures are atonic, absence, and myoclonic.
D. It is usually limited to children younger than two years of age.

67. Which of the following is characteristic of status epilepticus?

A. Seizures last for 10 minutes or more, without a lucid interval.
B. Seizure activity occurs multiple times within a 24-hour time frame.
C. There is the presence of an aura, and there are postictal periods.
D. Seizures are generalized tonic-clonic in nature.

68. Which of these medications is not commonly used in the treatment of epilepsy?

A. Carbamazepine
B. Phenytoin
C. Celecoxib
D. Benzodiazepines

69. A 26-year-old female is taking a walk when she has a sudden transient loss of consciousness. She has no significant past medical history. Which of the following best explains this presentation?

A. Syncope
B. Cerebrovascular accident
C. Transient ischemic attack
D. Seizure syndrome

70. A 25-year-old male has difficulty breathing. His respiratory rate is 40 cpm. He is anxious and restless with an SPO2 of 85% in-room oxygen. Part of your emergency care is to keep this patient's airway patent, commence assisted ventilation with a BVM, and give supplemental oxygen. Which of the following tenets prohibits you from performing endotracheal intubation?

A. Duty to act
B. Scope of practice
C. Standard of care
D. Civil law

71. You attended to a 43-year-old male who had a closed fracture to the right humerus following a fall from height. You were able to splint the limb and immobilize the patient during transfer to the receiving center. A few weeks later, the patient sues you for negligence. For the patient to do this, he must prove all except which of the following?

A. Causation
B. Breach of duty
C. Standard of care
D. Duty to act

72. Which of the following is an example of battery?

A. Threatening to use handcuffs on a patient with alcohol intoxication
B. Applying a cervical collar to an unconscious patient involved in an MVC
C. Splinting the broken limb of a conscious patient without consent
D. Forgetting to inspect the back of a patient with a gunshot injury to the abdomen

73. EMT M and his partner have just concluded their shift when an emergency call comes through the pager. There is no one available to answer the call, so they both agree to answer the call. Which of the following best describes their reason for doing so?

A. Duty to act
B. Beneficence
C. Veracity
D. Standard of care

74. You are attending to a 45-year-old female who experiences crushing chest pain, difficulty breathing, and anxiety. She had an episode of syncope just before you arrived. As you do a primary survey, the patient tells you she is fine and does not wish to go to the hospital for ECG and management. You are expected to do all except which of the following?

A. Assess the patient's alertness and orientation.
B. Explain the implication of the patient's refusal.
C. Document the patient's response.
D. Refer the patient to a psychologist for counseling

75. An EMT who has just attended to a 24-year-old male with multiple fractures following a motor vehicle collision describes the patient as "drunk" to the emergency nurse in the receiving center. This EMT has demonstrated which of the following?

A. Bias
B. Libel
C. Slander
D. Insensitivity

76. You respond to a call to attend to a 75-year-old female with apnea. On examination, her pulse is fast and thready and her respiratory rate is 6 cpm. The woman's caregiver says the woman has a DNR order. Which of the following responses is most appropriate?

A. Transport the patient to the ER.
B. Commence BVM ventilation.
C. Request the DNR certificate.
D. Give IV morphine.

77. The Health Insurance Portability and Accountability Act (HIPAA) prevents EMTs from doing all except which of the following?

A. Sharing patients' information with friends
B. Sharing patients' information with spouses
C. Sharing patients' information with other crew members
D. Sharing patients' information with the receiving nurse

78. You are attending to a 65-year-old male who just had a fainting episode. On examination, his pulse rate is full volume and rapid. His respiratory rate is 24 cpm. He tells you he is scheduled for a visit with his cardiologist in a week and is not interested in going to the ER. Which of the following ethical principles should guide your response to this patient?

A. Veracity
B. Autonomy
C. Fidelity
D. Beneficence

79. As a leader of your response team, you are expected to do all except which of the following?

A. Encourage all team members to wash their hands after attending to patients.
B. Ask for input from team members.
C. Make all decisions in the field.
D. Collect information from witnesses.

80. You are lifting a 35-year-old male victim of a motor vehicle crash from the ground to the stretcher. Which of the following statements is incorrect?

A. At least two people should lift this patient.
B. Your spine should be locked as you lift.
C. You should keep the patient close to your body as you lift.
D. You should engage the muscles in your back as you lift.

81. Which of the following is most appropriate in carrying a 45-year-old male who is conscious and alert, with no suspected injury to the spine?

A. Stretcher
B. Backboard
C. Stair chair
D. Reeves sleeve

82. Which of the following is not an indication for quickly moving a patient out of an environment?

A. Shock
B. Fire
C. Radiation
D. Spinal injury

83. You are about to do an emergency move on a 35-year-old male involved in a motor vehicle crash. This patient is caught underneath a vehicle. Which of the following statements is false?

A. You should pull the patient along the long axis of his body.
B. You should tug at the collar of the patient's shirt.
C. You should use the direct ground lift.
D. You should drag the patient on a blanket.

84. Which of the following positions is most appropriate for a 43-year-old male who experiences difficulty breathing, chest pain, anxiety, cough, and cyanosis?

A. Supine position
B. Fowler's position
C. Trendelenburg position
D. Left lateral position

85. Your team is responding to a mass casualty incident where victims have been exposed to radiologic agents. Which of the following precautions is not useful in protecting you and your team from exposure?

A. Wearing Level A gear
B. Reducing the duration of exposure
C. Decontaminating with hypochlorite solution
D. Shielding the source of exposure

86. Which of the following is the third-leading cause of death in all age groups and the leading cause of death and disability in the United States among young adults (up to 44 years old) and children?

A. Trauma
B. Cancer
C. Drug abuse
D. Gunshot

87. Body tissues are occasionally exposed to energy levels. Which of the following statements is correct about the mechanism of energy levels on body tissues?

A. Energy levels are beyond the body's tolerance.
B. Energy levels are repeatedly hitting the body.
C. Energy levels come from a high-velocity object.
D. Energy levels come from an object bigger than the individual.

88. A 14-year-old male was hit by a car while riding his bicycle. All except which of the following are useful in assessing this patient?

A. The seating position of the patient
B. The form of restraint available and if it was used
C. The type of vehicle
D. The patient's level of consciousness of before the accident

89. A patient was in a motor vehicle collision. On examination, you notice a whiplash injury, which will require a neck collar for stabilization. Which of the following collisions is likely?

A. Frontal collision
B. Rear-end collision
C. Lateral collision
D. Rollover collision

90. A 55-year-old female had a domestic accident. On examination, the injury is not completely a penetrating injury but is a cavitation. The patient must have suffered from which form of penetrating injury?

A. Low velocity
B. Medium velocity
C. High velocity
D. Both B and C

91. A patient fell from a height three times his height. In considering the extent of internal injuries sustained, all except which of the following mechanical factors should be considered?

A. Height of the fall
B. Type of surface the man fell on
C. Medical causes of the fall
D. Part of the man's body that hit the surface first

92. From the above case study, which factor should you not consider in measuring the severity of the injury from the fall?

A. Height of the fall
B. Underlying medical causes before the fall
C. Presence of internal injuries from the fall
D. Family history of falls

93. In eliciting a history from a patient who suffered a blast injury, you are informed that the patient was thrown against the object of injury. What phase of blast injury is likely?

A. Primary phase
B. Secondary phase
C. Tertiary phase
D. None of the above

94. In accessing a patient with trauma, which of the following will you likely not consider?

A. Mechanism of injury
B. General impression of the patient
C. Priority determination
D. Time of injury

95. You are evacuating a victim of trauma with a significant mechanism of injury. En route to the hospital, what form of secondary assessment will you perform on the patient?

A. Rapid examination
B. Detailed examination
C. Rapid trauma examination
D. Focused examination

96. In assessing and managing trauma patients, all except which of the following general ideas are correct?

A. Hospitals/operating rooms provide better and holistic care for serious patients.
B. Achieving balanced care for life-threatening injuries and transport of severely injured patients is vital.
C. Identifying seriously injured patients is imperative.
D. Only initial assessment decisions, without MOI determination, are important in actual patient care.

97. Your friend has a bruise following a minor fall down the stairs. Which of the following is false regarding your friend's skin?

A. The epidermis will remain intact.
B. Cells and blood vessels within the dermis will be damaged.
C. There will be swelling and pain at the site of the injury.
D. There will not be any discoloration at the site.

98. A 45-year-old driver was involved in a head-on collision on his way to work. He is comatose and has severe traumatic brain injuries. An assessment of subdural hematoma is made. Which of the following is least likely to occur in this man?

A. Collection of blood beneath the scalp
B. Damaged cerebral blood vessels
C. An insignificant amount of tissue damage compared to a contusion
D. Massive blood loss, up to a liter or more

99. On your way home from work, you witness an accident where a car, on hitting a bystander, rolls over the person's thighs and lower abdomen. All except which of the following pathological processes are likely to occur?

A. Rupture of internal organs
B. Preserved bony integrity
C. Severe internal bleeding
D. Hypoperfusion or shock

100. If you were to manage the above patient, what unlikely step would you take if you suspect hypoperfusion or shock?

A. Respond to the shock by restricting IV fluid administration.
B. Treat the hypoperfusion.
C. Splint any swollen, painful, or deformed extremity.
D. Document all necessary findings on assessment.

101. A patient presents with the outermost layer of the skin of her left thigh damaged by shearing forces, with leakage of a small amount of blood. Which of the following soft tissue injuries is likely?

A. Contusion
B. Abrasion
C. Crush injury
D. Hematoma

102. Which of the following statements is not true about a laceration?

A. It is caused by the impact of forceful sharp objects.
B. It can be caused by a gunshot.
C. It is associated with severe bleeding.
D. It is associated with varying depth of skin breakage and damage.

103. A man was stabbed in the left hypochondriac region. There is severe internal bleeding and a visible stab wound at the back. Which of the following tissue injuries best describes this?

A. Avulsion
B. Crush injury
C. Puncture
D. Laceration

104. In the management of a patient with an open soft tissue injury of the right arm, which of the following is the least likely step you should take?

A. Ensure the wound is exposed.
B. Control the bleeding.
C. Administer high-concentration oxygen.
D. Apply a dry sterile dressing to the wound.

105. A 45-year-old female is rushed to the ER with a laceration in her abdomen and evisceration of her intestines. Which of the following treatment processes will likely not be beneficial to the woman?

A. Trying to replace her exposed organs
B. Covering the exposed organs with a sterile dressing
C. Moistening a sterile dressing with saline or sterile water before application
D. Flexing the patient's hip and knees if not injured

106. You are the ERT on duty, and you attend to a patient with a partially amputated left hand. Which of the following interventions is inappropriate?

A. Covering the amputated part with a sterile dressing
B. Completing the amputation
C. Immobilizing the amputated part to prevent further injury
D. Controlling bleeding if massive

107. What is the leading cause of death and disability for children and adults up to 45 years of age?

A. Soft tissue injury
B. Traumatic brain injury
C. Penetrating injury
D. Blast injury

108. Your team is called to a home where a 13-year-old male has fallen from a tree. When you arrive, the boy's mother is crying for you to help him. The boy is sitting under the tree, clutching his right arm, which is oddly positioned, and his sweatshirt and the surrounding grass are stained with blood. The boy is pale and crying. His pulse rate is 150 bpm with a respiratory rate of 32 cpm. What is the most likely cause of this presentation?

A. Hypovolemia from blood loss
B. Anxiety from the pain of injury
C. Cardiogenic shock
D. Psychogenic shock

109. A 2-year-old female has been vomiting and passing frequent loose stools for the past three days since attending a birthday party. Her mother says she has had a fever and has been weak since yesterday but suddenly stopped responding to her name this afternoon. The girl is lying in bed, conscious but lethargic, with a pulse rate of 200 bpm, respiratory rate of 48 cpm. What is the most likely cause of this presentation?

A. Poisoning
B. Hypovolemic shock from dehydration
C. Septic shock
D. Respiratory tract infection

110. You are performing CPR on a 5-year-old male who suddenly collapsed with grunting respirations and no pulse. Which of the following is essential to know about performing CPR?

A. Chest compressions should be administered at a rate of 120 per minute.
B. Compressions should depress half of the anterior-posterior diameter of the chest or half an inch in infants and one inch in children.
C. Chest compressions should be done on the sternum, not the ribs.
D. A compression-to-ventilation ratio of 30:1 is recommended.

111. You are called to a home in the suburbs where a 10-year-old female with sickle cell anemia who just returned from a summer camp developed difficulty breathing while playing outside. She complains of pain in both shoulders and her left ankle, which started the previous day. She is pale, with yellow eyes, a pulse rate of 112 bpm and a respiratory rate of 28 cpm. What is the most likely cause of this presentation?

A. Vaso-occlusive crisis
B. Fractures of the shoulder and ankle joints
C. Hypovolemia from dehydration
D. Anaphylaxis

112. A 5-year-old male experiences respiratory distress, wheezing, drooling, and muffled speech after a bee sting. What is the first step in the management of this patient?

A. Administer supplemental oxygen.
B. Perform abdominal thrusts.
C. Give five rapid back blows.
D. Assist the patient in using an epinephrine injector.

113. A 2-year-old male was found in respiratory distress. He is conscious but cyanotic. His skin is cold and clammy. On auscultation, no air exchange in lung zones is notable. Which intervention should you take?

A. Perform five back blows and chest thrusts.
B. Commence CPR.
C. Perform abdominal thrusts.
D. Give high-flow oxygen using a non-rebreather mask.

114. A 1-year-old male has a fever, barking cough and noisy breathing. His fever is worse at night, and he is irritable. He has a significant tracheal tug and inspiratory stridor at rest. His temperature is 38° C, and his respiratory rate is 40 breaths per minute. Which of the following is an appropriate intervention?

A. Give oral acetaminophen.
B. Administer humidified oxygen.
C. Give IV corticosteroid.
D. Administer IV adrenaline.

115. A 5-year-old male has a history of fever, sore throat, and inability to swallow. He is sitting upright, neck hyperextended, jaw thrust forward, and mouth open. He has inspiratory stridor, cyanosis, and subcostal retractions. His temperature is 40° C, and his respiration is 46 breaths per minute. Which of the following is an appropriate intervention?

A. Lay the patient in the supine position.
B. Use a spatula to examine the patient's throat.
C. Administer blow-by oxygen while making transport arrangements for emergency care.
D. Administer oxygen via nasal prongs.

116. Which of the following statements is false regarding the APGAR score?

A. It is a quick way to assess a newborn infant.
B. It is made up of five components.
C. Scores range from 0 to 2 for each component.
D. A composite score is computed at 1 and 7 minutes.

117. You and your partner have just responded to a home birth. In the fifth minute of life, the female neonate is completely pink and has a heart rate of 108 bpm. You consider her respiratory efforts to be adequate. She maintains her limbs in a flexed position and grimaces on stimulation. What is the infant's APGAR score?

A. 9
B. 10
C. 8
D. 7

118. A 9-year-old male is seen coughing with difficulty breathing. On examination, he is breathing through pursed lips and uses accessory muscles for respiration. You also note that he is wheezing. Which of the following is not an appropriate intervention?

A. Assist the patient with his prescribed metered-dose inhaler.
B. Assist the patient with his prescribed epinephrine injection.
C. Place the patient in a comfortable position.
D. Administer oxygen if the boy's saturation levels are low.

119. You are called to see a 3-year-old child who has had a high-grade fever in the past two days with vomiting that has progressively worsened. On examination, you notice the child is lethargic and has red spots across his limbs, face, and back, with some tenderness around his neck. Which of the following should you do?

A. Wear respiratory protection.
B. Manage the child for diarrhea.
C. Use a tepid sponge on the child.
D. Advise the parents to take their child for a measles vaccination.

120. A 6-year-old child is brought in by his parents after he accidentally spilled hot water from a kettle on himself. On examination, you notice burn wounds throughout his two lower limbs and his genital area. What is the percentage of burn wounds following the Wallace rule?

A. 32%
B. 33%
C. 34%
D. 36%

Test 1: Answers and Explanations

1. (D) Carry out an initial assessment looking for any immediate threats to life.
Assessing a patient allows you to develop a plan of action for the patient's management. This includes getting an initial impression as you arrive on the scene and assessing vital signs for airway, breathing, and respiration.

2. (D) Dehydration
Frequent stooling and vomiting for a week means the patient has lost a lot of electrolytes. He is at risk for hypovolemic shock.

3. (A) The heart
In hypovolemia, the body draws blood from the peripheral circulation and preserves it for the vital organs, the most important organ being the heart.

4. (A) Placing her in a supine position and administering supplemental oxygen
The patient is most likely hypovolemic. Placing her in a supine position and commencing oxygen will reduce the burden of her heart pumping oxygenated blood to her brain. The patient should then be transported to a hospital.

5. (B) Trauma to his cervical spine
Trauma to the cervical spine can cause widespread vasodilation, leading to neurogenic shock.

6. (D) Apply a tourniquet proximal to the injury and leave the shard in.
A tourniquet could be applied proximal to the wound. When an object is impaled in any of the extremities, it is best to leave the object in, as it may be acting as a tamponade for damaged blood vessels.

7. (A) Wrapping your bandage distal to the slit
Your tourniquet should be applied proximal to the wound to stop the exsanguination of damaged blood vessels.

8. (A) Place the patient in a comfortable position, administer oxygen, and transport her quickly to a hospital.
Myocardial infarction and angina should be managed similarly because it is difficult to exclusively make a diagnosis of one or the other in the field.

9. (A) Aortic dissection
Stabbing chest pain with unequal pulses is a classic feature of aortic dissection.

10. (C) Cardiogenic shock
Pulmonary edema may occur in patients with cardiogenic shock who then present with shortness of breath, crackles, and decreased saturation in addition to symptoms of cardiogenic shock.

11. (D) 30 chest compressions followed by 2 rescue breaths
Thirty chest compressions to two rescue breaths are the standard according to AHA guidelines.

12. (D) Chest compressions and artificial ventilation should be stopped when shocks are being delivered.
When shocks are to be delivered, the patient should be cleared.

13. (A) Rush the patient to the hospital while your coresponders administer CPR.
This should not be part of the treatment regimen. If you are transporting a conscious patient with chest pain who becomes unconscious, you should stop the vehicle and start resuscitation with CPR and AED.

14. (B) Allow as much ventilation as possible.
Option B is not correct according to AHA guidelines. Ventilations in high-quality CPR should be done in a ratio of 30 compressions to 2 breaths.

15. (D) If breathing is not present but pulse is felt, start CPR with cycles of 30 chest compressions and three breaths.
Option D is not part of an emergency medical responder's job. CPR is done as 30 chest compressions to two breaths if a patient has a pulse with abnormal or no breathing.

16. (C) Provide rescue breathing of 10 breaths/min; check pulse every two minutes and commence CPR if it is absent.
If a patient has a pulse but is not breathing, rescue breaths at a rate of 10 to 12 breaths per minute should be administered.

17. (D) Do a jaw thrust without head extension to open the airway.
For patients with a risk of cervical spine injury, a jaw thrust is preferred when administering oxygen, as it can be done with little or no movement of the spine.

18. (B) Start chest compressions immediately, giving 30 chest compressions followed by two breaths while waiting for an AED.

For patients in cardiac arrest, it is best to start CPR without delay while waiting for an AED if it is available.

19. (A) Commence supplementary oxygen and keep the patient warm.
HbSS patients can experience painful crises caused by lactate buildup from tissue hypoxia. Administering supplemental oxygen is beneficial.

20. (B) Apply a tourniquet proximal to the bite site.
Option B will be least beneficial for this patient. Applying a tourniquet to venomous bites is not beneficial in any way. Instead, it may lead to loss of limb, as it isolates the venom to that limb.

21. (D) Tissue respiration by uptake of CO_2
The functions of the respiratory system do not include tissue respiration by uptake of CO_2. Rather, the respiratory system expels CO_2. It helps filter toxins from circulation and aids in the homeostasis and metabolism of certain drugs and enzymes. The lungs have enzymes that aid the metabolism of xenobiotics. Drugs that can be metabolized in the lungs include propofol, salmeterol, fluticasone, and budesonide. The lungs also support the conversion of ACE I to ACE II, a key enzyme in the regulation of blood pressure.

22. (B) Jaw thrust
Tilting the head or otherwise moving the neck is contraindicated in a patient with a possible cervical spine injury, but maintaining an airway and ventilation is a greater priority. If the patient has a suspected cervical injury, the jaw-thrust maneuver is used instead of the head-tilt/chin-lift maneuver.

23. (D) Administer oxygen.
The most likely cause of sudden onset dyspnea, unilateral leg swelling, and calf pain after a long flight is pulmonary embolism. A high index of suspicion is needed to make a diagnosis. The patient will benefit from supplemental oxygen or ventilation to maintain adequate oxygen saturation. Treatment is with anticoagulants and, sometimes, clot dissolution with systemic or catheter-directed thrombolysis and surgical removal. When anticoagulation is contraindicated, an inferior vena cava filter should be placed.

24. (D) Trachea
The trachea is part of the lower (not upper) airway. The upper airway serves as a conduit for gaseous exchange. It consists of the nostrils, mouth, nasopharynx, pharynx, and larynx. Combined, they work to not only channel air in and out of the body but to warm, humidify, and filter it as well.

25. (D) Inspiration produces a slight negative pressure inside the thoracic cavity.
At inspiration, the chest cavity increases in size as the diaphragm moves downward, and the ribs are pulled outward by the intercostal muscles. This produces a slight negative pressure inside the cavity, causing the lungs to expand and draw air in. This is the inspiratory phase of ventilation.

26. (D) Bronchioles
The lower airway begins at the level of the vocal cords and includes the trachea, main bronchi, and bronchioles, terminating in the alveoli. Inside the lungs are the bronchi, bronchioles, and alveoli.

27. (B) Increased carbon dioxide saturation in the blood
Chemoreceptors, found primarily in the brain stem, detect levels of carbon dioxide and oxygen. They send signals to the brain, which, in turn, trigger an increase or decrease in the work of breathing. The brain is more sensitive to changes in CO_2 concentration. Patients who retain CO_2 all the time, such as those with chronic obstructive pulmonary disease (COPD), lose their ability to sense that gas. This makes them depend on the hypoxic drive to control their respiration.

28. (A) Respiratory distress
The patient is compensating for hypoxia by breathing faster and harder, leading to respiratory distress. If the compensatory mechanisms do not maintain adequate oxygen or carbon dioxide levels, the patient's well-being will begin to deteriorate. Failure in compensatory mechanisms causes CO_2 buildup and mental status changes, which cause respiratory failure. If left untreated, respiratory failure deteriorates to respiratory arrest, and cardiac arrest soon follows.

29. (B) Reassure the patient and perform a secondary assessment.
The patient does not require supplemental oxygen, as saturation levels are good. Tachypnea, tachycardia, and elevated blood pressure may be a result of panic and agitation from the incident, hence the need to calm the patient down and reassess her. Antihypertensives are not indicated, and breathing into a paper bag is inappropriate for this level of care.

30. (A) Commence BVM ventilation.
The patient is hypoxic and lapsing into unconsciousness; this is an indicator of imminent respiratory failure. Delivering manual ventilation with a bag and mask will prevent further deterioration of her physical state. A non-rebreather mask is used in a hypoxic patient with adequate respiratory effort. Cardiopulmonary resuscitation is not indicated in this scenario. A corticosteroid inhaler will not help improve saturation levels.

31. (C) Asthma
Individuals with atopy have an increased risk of developing asthma. This is because they form IgE antibodies to common allergens. Atopy is the strongest risk factor in the development of asthma. The patient has allergic rhinitis and dermatitis, which indicates atopy. Bronchiolitis may present with wheezing and cough; however, a slight fever is common. Bronchiectasis presents with a daily cough with copious amounts of phlegm over months or years. Cystic fibrosis causes chronic persistent cough and thick sputum production.

32. (D) All of the above
In asthma, there is airway inflammation and hyperresponsiveness to already sensitized allergens. This causes airflow limitation, respiratory symptoms, and subsequent chronicity of asthma. Pathological changes in some patients with asthma include fibrosis of the sub-basement layer, hypersecretion of mucus, hypertrophy of smooth muscles, neovascularization, and injury to epithelial cells.

33. (A) Chest rises and falls with each ventilation.
An EMT is giving adequate artificial ventilation to a patient when there is a chest rise and fall with each ventilation. The sufficient rate for ventilation in adults is 10 to 12 times per minute, and 12 to 20 times per minute for children and infants. Improvement of cyanosis and heart rate returning to normal are all indicators of successful artificial ventilation.

34. (C) 300 mmHg
Suction devices should be inspected regularly. A properly functioning suction unit with a gauge produces a 300 mmHg vacuum. Battery-operated suction units should have a charged battery. There are various types of suction units, which include manual, mounted, and portable. If there is no gauge available in a suction unit, allow the suction tubing to begin suctioning on the finger, then turn the suction unit off. If the tubing stays attached, then suction is adequate.

35. (A) Nasopharyngeal airway
Nasopharyngeal airways are indicated when a patient is semiconscious and may have a gag reflex like the patient in the scenario described in this question. Airway devices include oral airway devices and nasopharyngeal airway devices, which are also called nasal trumpets. Airway adjuncts are important in improving the success rate of basic airway procedures. They open up the airway, aiding spontaneous respiration or BVM ventilation. In most patients with unconsciousness or a reduced level of consciousness, there is a risk of the tongue falling back into the posterior pharynx and occluding the upper airway. A nasopharyngeal airway is therefore an important tool because it stents the airway open. The laryngeal mask airway is a supraglottic airway device used to keep the upper airway open in cases of difficult airway or failed endotracheal intubation. A non-rebreather mask is used for oxygen delivery.

36. (C) Insert an oropharyngeal airway and begin ventilation.
Opioids like heroin and morphine cause altered mental states and depress the respiratory drive. Depression of the respiratory drive causes slow, shallow respirations, which can deteriorate to respiratory arrest. For this patient, you should insert an oropharyngeal airway to control the airway, perform a head-tilt/chin-lift maneuver, and begin ventilation with a BVM and oxygen. Performing CPR and placing the patient in the left recumbent position will not improve respiratory depression. A non-rebreather mask should be used in a patient who is hypoxic but can make an adequate respiratory effort.

37. (A) Help the patient into a comfortable position and administer supplemental oxygen.
This patient is suffering from secondary spontaneous pneumothorax. For this patient, oxygen supplementation is necessary. The patient has risk factors associated with pneumothorax. It can occur after heavy lifting, a history of asthma, and significant smoking. Necessary arrangements for emergency transport should also be made. The patient does not have an acute asthma exacerbation; hence a rescue inhaler is not useful. Breathing into a paper bag will not help improve oxygen saturation. Oral acetaminophen is not beneficial in this situation.

38. (C) Emphysema
There is a history of significant smoking; chronic cough; wheezing; thin appearance; red, flushed skin; and reduced SaO_2. Hence, the case scenario is suggestive of COPD (emphysema). Chronic bronchitis is unlikely because even though the symptoms may overlap, they usually present with symptoms of right-sided heart failure (bilateral pedal edema, increased jugular venous pressure and cyanosis). Hence the term "blue bloater" in chronic bronchitis. Bronchial asthma presents with nocturnal cough and chest tightness.

39. (A) Destruction of lung parenchyma, leading to loss of elastic recoil and alveolar destruction
The pathophysiology of emphysema is the destruction of the alveolar wall and irreversible enlargement of airspaces distal to terminal bronchiole. Loss of elastic recoil, alveolar septa destruction, and radial airway traction in emphysema increase the tendency for the airway to collapse. Hyperinflation of the lungs, airflow limitation, and air trapping follow. Hypersensitive airway responsiveness is seen in asthma. Viral lung infection is not implied in the pathophysiology of emphysema. The collapse of lung tissue and loss of volume is seen in atelectasis.

40. (C) Hyperventilation
Patients with emphysema are called pink puffers due to hyperventilation. Destruction of the pulmonary capillary bed and alveolar septa in emphysema reduces oxygenation of the blood. Compensatory responses of the body include lowering of cardiac output and hyperventilation. This ventilation-perfusion mismatch relatively limits blood flow through the lungs. Because of reduced cardiac output, the rest of the body suffers from tissue hypoxia and pulmonary cachexia. These patients eventually develop muscle wasting.

41. (C) Give supplemental oxygen using a Venturi mask.
The case scenario is that of pneumonia in a patient with chronic bronchitis. In patients with COPD, giving low-flow oxygen using a Venturi mask is most helpful, as this will improve oxygen saturation without risk of worsening respiratory acidosis. The risk of respiratory acidosis in patients with COPD is markedly increased with the use of high-flow oxygen. This makes use of high-flow oxygen with a non-rebreather mask erroneous. Determining the patient's blood pressure will not help. A rescue bronchodilator inhalation could be helpful, but only after adequate measures have been taken to improve the patient's oxygen saturation.

42. (D) 24%–60%
The Venturi mask is a low-flow mask. It delivers 24%–60% oxygen at different flow rates. A Venturi mask is important in oxygen delivery to patients with COPD, as it supplies low-flow oxygen and reduces the risk of respiratory acidosis in this group of patients.

43. (D) Give the patient inhaled bronchodilators using a metered-dose inhaler.
The case scenario is acute asthmatic exacerbation with metabolic skin change. An inhaled bronchodilator is the most appropriate intervention. Oral corticosteroids are not contraindicated, and injectable epinephrine may not help as it is not allergen triggered. And even though administering oxygen may be beneficial, it is most important to first relieve the patient's bronchospasms.

44. (A) Give the patient an epinephrine injection.
The history of this patient points to a peanut butter allergy, which led to anaphylaxis. The physical symptoms are also in keeping with this diagnosis; thus, the patient will benefit most from an epinephrine injection. Supplemental oxygen may also be required depending on oxygen saturation.

45. (C) Administer low-flow oxygen via nasal cannula.
This is a case of emphysema. As the patient is conscious and able to breathe by himself, a bag and mask are unnecessary. He will require low-flow oxygen via a nasal cannula to optimize his saturation.

46. (A) Insert an oropharyngeal airway.
The first thing to do is to secure her airway with an oropharyngeal airway device, after which supplemental oxygen can be administered via BVM. The patient is unconscious, so a nasal cannula should not be used to deliver oxygen.

47. (A) Help the patient into a comfortable position.
The scenario is suggestive of spontaneous pneumothorax, so management will include helping the patient into a comfortable position and administering supplemental oxygen. There is no indication of asthma in the stem; thus, an inhaler is not necessary. As the patient is conscious and able to breathe by himself, a BVM will be an inappropriate method for delivering supplemental oxygen. A nasal cannula or non-rebreather mask will be more appropriate for this patient.

48. (A) Assist the patient with her prescribed multidose inhaler.
This patient is suffering from an asthma attack. The most important intervention is to assist her with her prescribed inhaler. Breathing into a paper bag will worsen her saturation. Considering the level of distress she is in, administering high-flow oxygen would be ideal; however, commencing BVM ventilation is unnecessary, as she is conscious.

49. (C) Croup
The child's age, raspy cough, and stridor are features of croup. Management will include placing the child in a comfortable position and administering humidified oxygen.

50. (D) Administer low-flow oxygen via a nasal cannula.
The most likely diagnosis here is pneumonia. As the patient is conscious and able to breathe by herself, providing supplemental oxygen via a nasal cannula will suffice. Assisting the patient into a comfortable position will not do much for her symptoms.

51. (B) Pulmonary embolism
A combination of chest pain, recent long-distance flight, smoking, and localized wheeze points to pulmonary embolism. A patient with COPD or asthma will likely have experienced these symptoms previously and will probably have an inhaler. Also look out for other physical symptoms, like barrel chest, dusky skin, and breathing through pursed lips. In a patient with bronchopneumonia, expected symptoms will include fever and flu-like symptoms and a productive cough.

52. (B) Administer oxygen to the patient via a nasal cannula.
Administering oxygen via a nasal cannula is the safest line of action to take for this patient. Although his symptoms are suggestive of a panic attack, he may also be suffering from a pulmonary embolism; thus, breathing into a paper bag may do more harm than good.

53. (C) Assist the patient in taking his prescribed nitroglycerin tablet.
This man is suffering from acute coronary syndrome. Assist him with his prescribed nitroglycerin tablet while transporting him as quickly and safely as possible to the nearest cardiac hospital. A further history may be taken if time permits after the patient has been stabilized and is being transported to a hospital. You are not authorized to give the patient any ulcer medication, even if it has been prescribed.

54. (A) Administer oxygen via a nasal cannula.
Supplemental oxygen will be beneficial to this patient to improve his saturation. You could also place him in a full sitting position with his feet dangling, as this can improve his blood pressure while he is being transported. Further assessment before transportation will only delay the patient's management.

55. (B) Aortic dissection
Aortic dissection is caused by a sudden rupture of an aortic aneurysm. Symptoms include those detailed in this question. This patient should be placed in a supine position if possible, and oxygen saturation and body temperature should be maintained. Acute coronary syndrome will usually present as chest pressure or heaviness, which radiates to the neck, shoulder, back, or jaw. Look out for signs of an infective process, fever, and hypotension in a patient with septic shock. Tension pneumothorax will present with more dramatic respiratory signs, including tracheal deviation and a hyperresonant thorax on percussion.

56. (B) Administer supplemental oxygen.
This patient's history is suggestive of sepsis. Administering supplemental oxygen to improve saturation will be most beneficial. You are not authorized to prescribe antidiarrheal medication, and a secondary assessment is not necessary at the moment. Sitting the patient upright in bed will not improve her condition in any way.

57. (C) For adults, space ventilation so that three breaths are delivered after every 20 compressions.
This statement is incorrect. The correct CPR protocol is to deliver two breaths after every 30 chest compressions in adult patients. Aim to deliver at least 100 chest compressions each minute, with a compression depth of at least two inches, allowing for full chest recoil after each compression. In adults, enough ventilation should be administered to make the chest visibly rise.

58. (D) Gastrointestinal bleeding
A history of peptic ulcer disease, binge drinking, and melena stool are features of gastrointestinal bleeding. Alcohol further erodes the gastric lining and may precipitate gastrointestinal bleeding in persons with peptic ulcer disease. This bleeding may present clinically as hematemesis; vomiting of blood; or melena, the passage of altered blood in the stool.

59. (B) Check for a carotid pulse, begin CPR, apply AED pads.
This is the most appropriate sequence of management for this patient. A carotid pulse may be present, so the patient will require only artificial ventilation. However, if a carotid pulse is absent, CPR should be performed before applying AED pads, as studies have shown that there is an increased rate of resuscitation when CPR is performed for 1.5 to 3 minutes before defibrillation.

60. (C) Sickled cells have a longer life span and more oxygen-carrying capacity.
Option C is false. Sickled cells have less oxygen-carrying capacity and a shorter life span than normal red blood cells. Sickle cell disease occurs due to a mutated form of hemoglobin, hemoglobin S. This mutation causes red blood cells to become fragile and sickled in shape.

61. (A) Vaso-occlusive crisis
There should be a high risk of suspicion of sickle cell crisis in a child presenting with chest pain, jaundice, and swelling of the limbs, especially as his parents are both carriers of the sickling gene. Hemophilia will present at a much earlier age in males with a history of spontaneous hemorrhage or hemorrhage that is disproportionate to trauma. There will also be a family history of bleeding disorders. Patients with Dubin-Johnson syndrome will have jaundice without the classic limb and chest pain.

62. (A) Facial droop – Patients can show their teeth.
Facial droop is tested by having patients smile or show their teeth. Both sides of the face move equally in a normal patient.

63. (B) Basilar artery
Occlusion of the basilar arteries affects both cerebral hemispheres, so symptoms are seen on both sides of the body.

64. (C) Simple partial seizure
In a simple partial seizure, the pattern of symptoms is limited to the area of the brain with abnormal neural activity. Unlike in complex partial seizures, there is no impairment of consciousness.

65. (C) There is no mental retardation.
Option A is incorrect. West syndrome is an epilepsy syndrome characterized by the triad of infantile spasm, mental retardation, and an EEG pattern known as hypsarrhythmia. Most patients with West syndrome have some degree of developmental delay.

66. (D) It is usually limited to children younger than two years of age.
This statement is false. Lennox-Gastaut syndrome usually develops in children between one to eight years of age. It is also known as childhood epileptic encephalopathy. It is a childhood epilepsy syndrome characterized by multiple seizure types, mental retardation or regression, and abnormal electroencephalography findings.

67. (B) Seizure activity occurs multiple times within a 24-hour time frame.
This is referred to as acute repetitive seizures or cluster seizures.

68. (C) Celecoxib
Celecoxib is a nonsteroidal anti-inflammatory medication used for the treatment of pain, fever, and swelling caused by arthritis. Unlike the other medications listed, it has no antiseizure activity. On the contrary, it has convulsant/epileptogenic properties and may precipitate a seizure.

69. (A) Syncope
Syncope is a transient loss of consciousness that occurs due to a temporary loss of blood to the brain. It usually occurs when the patient is upright. Consciousness is regained when the person becomes horizontal. It can be caused by an array of conditions that may be cardiac- or noncardiac-related and may indicate a more serious underlying condition.

70. (B) Scope of practice
The scope of practice is created and enforced by state laws and defines the procedures and type of emergency care that can be given by an EMT. For example, according to the scope of practice, an EMT can perform BVM ventilation but cannot perform endotracheal intubation. Option A is incorrect because the duty to act means that EMTs are responsible for performing their duties to the highest standard as stated by the scope of practice. Option C is incorrect because the standard of care is the protocol used in performing certain procedures. It means that the way a procedure is performed by an EMT in a particular situation is the way it should be performed by another EMT in a similar situation.

71. (C) Standard of care
Negligence/malpractice is defined as a failure to perform duty. The following four elements are involved in negligence:
Duty to act – There must be evidence that the health worker did not fulfill the duty owed to the patient.
Breach of duty – There must be evidence that the health worker did not fulfill their obligation by performing as a reasonable health worker would perform in similar situations.
Causation – There must be a correlation between harm done to the patient and the health worker's breach of duty.
Harm/injury – There must be evidence of damage done by breach of duty.

72. (C) Splinting the broken limb of a conscious patient without consent.
This is an example of battery. Battery occurs when a health worker touches a patient or performs a procedure on a patient without consent. Implied or express consent must first be obtained. Option A describes assault; Option B describes duty to act; Option D describes negligence.

73. (B) Beneficence
The ethical principle of beneficence means that the health worker is expected to act in the best interest of a patient. Option A, duty to act, is incorrect because this call came after the shift. The EMTs are therefore not obligated to answer the call. Option C is incorrect because the ethical principle of veracity focuses on truthfulness and transparency in communicating with patients. Option D is incorrect because the standard of care is the protocol used in performing certain procedures.

74. (D) Refer the patient to a psychologist for counseling.
Referral to a psychologist is beyond the scope of practice of an EMT. Adults have the right to autonomy, provided they are fully capable and can understand the implications of accepting/refusing care. The EMT must first assess this patient's alertness and consciousness, explain the implication of refusing/accepting care, and assess likely factors that can impair the patient's judgment. Then the patient's refusal must be documented and her signature given for legal proof.

75. (C) Slander
In slander, an oral statement is made to tarnish someone's character. Slander is similar to libel; however, in libel, the statement is written. In this case, rather than make a subjective claim that the patient is drunk and was driving under the influence of alcohol, it is safer to report objective signs, like saying the patient has slurred speech or the patient was unsteady and had breath that smelled like alcohol. Whether or not the patient drove under the influence of alcohol will be decided by objective laboratory tests.

76. (C) Request the DNR certificate.
A DNR order is an advance directive that prohibits resuscitation in patients who request it. However, although resuscitation is prohibited, other supportive measures are given. In this patient, the EMT must first request the DNR certificate for confirmation. If this is not available, resuscitation must be commenced. If the DNR certificate is available, the patient should be transported to the receiving center. Option D is incorrect because IV morphine will worsen the patient's respiratory effort. Moreover, the administration of IV morphine is beyond an EMT's scope of practice.

77. (D) Sharing patients' information with the receiving nurse
The Health Insurance Portability and Accountability Act (HIPAA) prohibits health workers from sharing patients' health information with anyone who is not a member of the managing team. These include family, relatives, friends, crew members, and even health professionals who are not managing the patient. Sharing patients' information with the receiving nurse is appropriate, per HIPAA.

78. (B) Autonomy
The ethical principle of autonomy means that patients have the final say in the way they receive treatment. The principle of autonomy works with informed consent. Patients must be educated on their condition and the indications of the treatment provided, including the side effects and complications.

79. (C) Make all decisions in the field.
Although team leaders are responsible for overseeing the progress of their team, they do not have to make all the decisions in order for this to happen. Asking for input from team members, delegating tasks, and seeking feedback increase the success of response teams.

80. (D) You should engage the muscles in your back as you lift.
This statement is incorrect because the power to lift should come from the muscles in the legs, arms, and shoulders, not the back. The spine should be locked, and the muscles in the back should be relaxed. To avoid sprain and other soft tissue injuries to the lower back, do not bend the waist.

81. (C) Stair chair
The stair chair is the preferred device for carrying a conscious patient down the stairs. Unconscious patients and patients with spinal injuries should be moved on a stretcher. It is important to immobilize patients with suspected spinal injuries and fractures on a backboard.

82. (D) Spinal injury
Patients with a spinal injury must be stabilized before they are moved, as long as they are not in a life-threatening condition and the environment does not threaten their safety. Indications for urgently moving a patient include the presence of fire, explosives, radiation, and other hazardous material in the patient's environment; the patient is blocking access to other patients in life-threatening conditions; the presence of an immediate threat to the patient; the presence of life-threatening conditions, like apnea, shock, or altered sensorium; or the EMT is unable to protect the patient from hazards in the current environment.

83. (C) You should use the direct ground lift.
This statement is false, as this patient has suspected spinal injuries. The direct ground lift is used to move only patients without suspected spinal injuries. To protect the spine, you can move the patient by tugging at the collar of his shirt, placing him on a blanket and tugging the blanket, or dragging the patient by his forearms. In this case, you should anchor a hand underneath the patient's armpits and pull. In all the methods, the general rule is to pull the patient along the long axis of the body.

84. (B) Fowler's position
This patient has cardiac disease that prevents proper oxygenation of the lungs—probably a left ventricular heart failure or pulmonary edema. For comfort, the patient should be placed in the cardiac position/Fowler's position. The head of the bed should be elevated to about 40°. If this is not possible, the patient's head, neck, and chest should be propped up on pillows. This position allows gravitation of fluid to the bottom of the lungs (if the lungs are congested).

85. (C) Decontaminating with hypochlorite solution
This measure cannot protect you and your team from radiation exposure. Factors that can reduce the risk of exposure include wearing Level A gear for complete protection from the substance, cutting down the duration of exposure to the source, shielding the source of exposure, and increasing the distance between yourself and the radioactive material.

86. (A) Trauma
Trauma is the third-leading cause of death in all age groups in America. Each year, an estimated 25% of Americans are severely injured enough to seek medical attention, and about 23 to 28 million people are brought into the emergency department for traumatic injury. This includes all forms of traumatic injuries—chest, abdominal, head, and neck, as well as traumatic injuries of the ears, eyes, and genitalia.

87. (A) Energy levels are beyond the body's tolerance.
Option A is correct. Work is defined as a force acting over a distance. Any energy level that has a force greater than a body's restraint and tolerance will compress body tissues beyond their inherent limits, consequently resulting in the work that causes injury. All other options would be correct only if the object has a force greater than the body, which was not stated in the question.

88. (D) The patient's level of consciousness before the accident
Only the level of consciousness after the accident (not before) will be important in assessing severity. The severity of the injury will differ depending on the sitting position and whether a restraint, such as a seat belt, was available and used. Also, the type of vehicle will matter (for example, whether it had energy-absorbing structural devices to reduce impact).

89. (B) Rear-end collision
Whiplash injury refers to a sudden forceful thrust of the neck forward then backward. It is caused by a rear-end collision. While a frontal injury is suggestive of an airbag being deployed, a rollover is usually followed by ejection or partial ejection of the victim. Lateral collisions usually cause severe rib, shoulder, and one-sided arm injuries.

90. (D) Both B and C
A penetrating injury that affects only the primary site of penetration, such as a knife stab, is classified as low velocity. But with increased velocity, such as gunshots, the object carries with it pressure waves that cause surrounding impact. This is because the energy for an object to cause damage is increased four times with increasing velocity.

91. (C) Medical causes of the fall
The patient's underlying medical conditions, such as syncope, are factors to consider in examining the extent of the injury. But they are not a mechanical factor involved in the fall.

92. (D) Family history of falls
Since a family history of falls is not hereditary in this case, it is not a determining factor to consider.

93. (C) Tertiary phase
The mechanism of a blast injury has three phases—primary, secondary, and tertiary. Injuries sustained from the pressure waves of the blast are considered primary; those that occur by flying debris or particles are secondary. In the tertiary phase, the individual is thrown against an object.

94. (D) Time of injury
Unlike the other answer options, the time of injury has no direct impact on the severity of the trauma and, as such, will not be used in assessing the patient.

95. (B) Detailed examination
While rapid trauma examination involves a quick but effective way of looking out for life-threatening complications of injury, a detailed examination is a slower, more complete inspection that examines all parts of the body and is usually done en route to the hospital.

96. (D) Only initial assessment decisions, without MOI determination, are important in actual patient care.
Option D is incorrect. The MOI is key in determining the expected severity of the trauma, especially internal injuries. So, an initial assessment of patients without understanding the MOI is not correct in the assessment and management of trauma patients.

97. (D) There will not be any discoloration at the site.
This statement is false. Blood accumulation is typical of an inflammatory injury like a bruise, and it is the reason behind skin discoloration in response to an injury. There is epidermal infiltration and swelling, pain, and cellular and capillary endothelial damage within the dermis.

98. (C) An insignificant amount of tissue damage compared to contusion
This scenario is the least likely to occur in this patient. While a contusion results from leakage of blood from an injured or inflamed vessel, a hematoma seems worse with pooling of blood outside the vessel but within the damaged tissue. It is characterized by a larger amount of tissue damage compared to contusion.

99. (B) Preserved bony integrity
Preserved bony integrity is not likely to occur in this scenario. The case is an example of a crush injury, where part of a body is compressed or crushed between two objects, in this case between the car and the road. Preserved bony integrity, or innervation, following such a crush injury is unlikely compared to Options A, B, and C.

100. (A) Respond to the shock by restricting IV fluid administration.
This is an unlikely step when treating this patient if you suspect hypoperfusion or shock. Blood loss causes hypovolemia and compromises hemodynamic stability. Replacing blood and fluid volume by replacing with isotonic fluid is a principle of shock treatment as opposed to restricting IV fluid intake.

101. (B) Abrasion
All other options are examples of closed soft tissue injuries, usually with blood clots or pooling beneath the skin. An abrasion is characterized by damage of the outer layer of the skin, although it is superficial in most cases.

102. (B) It can be caused by a gunshot.
Option B is not true about lacerations. Lacerations are usually caused by sharp objects with forceful impact or cuts on the body. They are characterized by a break or tear of the skin with damage to soft tissues depending on depth, neurovascular compromise, and overall severity. Gunshots cause direct penetrating or puncture wounds or injuries.

103. (C) Puncture
A puncture or penetrating injury is likely in this scenario, usually caused by forceful sharp objects with a high-velocity application, such as stab wounds, and characterized by little or no external bleeding.

104. (C) Administer high-concentration oxygen.
Oxygen is the least likely step, as it is recommended in chest injuries only when respiratory activity is compromised. This is unlikely in this patient.

105. (A) Trying to replace her exposed organs
Trying to replace the patient's exposed organs is inappropriate, as it may contaminate the viscera and cause peritonitis.

106. (B) Completing the amputation
Completing the amputation will be detrimental, as the viability of the amputated part has to be ascertained by an orthopedic surgeon.

107. (B) Traumatic brain injury
In the United States approximately 1.6 million head injuries occur per year, with about 52,000 persons dying from traumatic brain injuries per year and 70,000 to 90,000 individuals left with neurological disabilities. In children, traumatic brain injuries are common from motor vehicle accidents either via automobile crashes or being struck down as pedestrians. Other causes are violence, child abuse, and falls. Soft tissue injuries and blast injuries are not as common as brain injuries.

108. (A) Hypovolemia from blood loss
The boy has most likely lost a lot of blood from a fracture of his right arm. This would account for the pallor, elevated pulse, and respiratory rate.

109. (B) Hypovolemic shock from dehydration
Vomiting and diarrhea are the most common causes of hypovolemic shock in children.

110. (C) Chest compressions should be done on the sternum, not the ribs.
Chest compressions should be done on the lower half of the sternum, depressing at least one-third of the AP diameter of the chest at the rate of 100 compressions per minute and with a compression-to-ventilation ratio of 30:2.

111. (A) Vaso-occlusive crisis
Vaso-occlusive crises are emergencies seen in sickle cell patients who experience bone pain. They usually occur when blood vessels are occluded by sickled cells, which leads to obstructed blood flow and tissue ischemia. Precipitating factors for the crisis include physical stress.

112. (D) Assist the patient in using an epinephrine injector.
Anaphylaxis is characterized by acute onset of stridor, hypotension, wheezing, and stridor. Diagnosis is clinical. Treatment is epinephrine. Beta-agonists are used to treat airway swelling and bronchospasm.

113. (A) Perform five back blows and chest thrusts.
Choking in an infant is usually caused by a foreign body placed in the mouth. If the airway obstruction is severe, then back blows, followed by chest thrusts, are administered to dislodge the object. Abdominal thrusts are performed on a conscious child. Commence cardiopulmonary resuscitation if a child is unconscious.

114. (B) Administer humidified oxygen.
The infant in this scenario has croup. A change in air temperature or humidity may reduce symptoms.

115. (C) Administer blow-by oxygen while making transport arrangements for emergency care.
From the history and presentation, epiglottitis is most likely. Dyspnea, tachypnea, and inspiratory stridor are present, causing the child to sit upright, lean forward, and hyperextend the neck with the jaw thrust forward and mouth open to enhance air exchange (tripod position). Lying supine will occlude the airway and may cause respiratory failure. In children with epiglottitis, the airway must be secured immediately. Examining the throat with a spatula will trigger laryngeal spasms and should be avoided until the airway is secured. Giving oxygen via nasal prongs will not improve the patient's symptoms.

116. (D) A composite score is computed at 1 and 7 minutes.
This statement is false regarding the APGAR score. Scores are usually assigned at the first and fifth minutes of neonatal life. Scores of 7 and above are considered normal.

117. (C) 8
Based on the APGAR scoring chart, the infant scores two points each for heart rate, respiratory effort, and color, and one point for muscle tone and reflex irritability, bringing her total score to eight.

118. (B) Assist the patient with his prescribed epinephrine injection.
Option B is not an appropriate intervention. This child has signs of an acute asthma attack; hence, he does not require an epinephrine injection. Arrangements should be made to transport him to an appropriate hospital immediately while notifying his parents en route.

119. (A) Wear respiratory protection.
This child's symptoms are highly suggestive of meningitis. This is a highly contagious condition, and as such, the EMT should wear respiratory protection. Prepare to manage this child's airway and ventilation if respiratory failure occurs, and transport quickly.

120. (C) 34%
A score of 16.5 is assigned for each burned lower limb, and a score of one is assigned for genital region burns in children, bringing the total estimate for this child to 34%.

Test 2: Questions

1. As an EMT, you can be involved with dead/dying patients. Which of the following methods is inappropriate in helping families cope with grief?

   A. Being mindful of religious beliefs
   B. Using open-ended questions
   C. Reassuring the families of the outcome of the patient
   D. Using silence to communicate

2. Which of the following is not a stage in the process of grief?

   A. Denial
   B. Bargaining
   C. Depression
   D. Regret

3. Which of the following is false about critical stress incident management?

   A. It helps workers exposed to secondary trauma.
   B. It should commence at the scene of the incident.
   C. Debriefing meetings are held no later than 72 hours after the event.
   D. Meetings are supervised by a psychologist.

4. You and your partner responded to a call from a woman with anaphylaxis from bee stings. You both decide she needs an immediate epinephrine injection and decide to call medical control through a radio transmitter. Which of the following is not a principle of reporting this patient's case over the radio?

   A. Avoid using codes.
   B. Avoid saying "yes" or "no."
   C. Mention only the patient's first name.
   D. Use a monotone voice.

5. Which of the following actions is not a component of preassignment operations?

   A. Inspecting the hood of the ambulance
   B. Inspecting the batteries in the AED
   C. Charging the portable suction equipment
   D. Using seat belts when driving

6. Which of the following is unlikely to increase the risk of your ambulance crashing en route to the incident location?

A. Using air horns
B. Using red lights
C. Using headlights
D. Using escort vehicles

7. You are the driver in an ambulance headed to an incident location. At an intersection, the traffic light changes from green to yellow. Which of the following responses is most appropriate?

A. Turn on the airhorn to notify other drivers that you will be moving.
B. Drive through the intersection before the light turns red.
C. Prepare to maneuver the vehicle.
D. Slow down and stop if the light turns red.

8. In which of the following cases is the use of escorts and multiple ambulances acceptable?

A. Mass casualties
B. Unfamiliar routes
C. Newly employed EMT
D. Government officials

9. To reduce the risk of crashes of escorts and multiple ambulances, which of the following guidelines is unnecessary?

A. Avoiding red lights
B. Using sirens
C. Driving at a safe distance from one another
D. Obeying traffic lights

10. Which of the following is false about albuterol?

A. It reduces the secretion of mucus plugs.
B. It should be used with caution in patients with thyroid disease.
C. It is a category C drug.
D. It should be given as oral tablets.

11. You have just given 0.3 mg of IM epinephrine to a patient with anaphylaxis. Which of the following symptoms is epinephrine used for?

A. Urticaria
B. Diarrhea
C. Wheezing
D. Nausea

12. You have just administered nitroglycerin to a patient with shortness of breath and crushing chest pain from myocardial infarction. You must monitor the patient for all except which of the following side effects?

A. Syncope
B. Headache
C. Urticaria
D. Blurred vision

13. An EMT is permitted to administer all except which of the following drugs?

A. Activated charcoal
B. Aspirin
C. Albuterol
D. Heparin

14. Activated charcoal is useful in treating all except which of the following types of poisoning?

A. Acetaminophen
B. Digoxin
C. Theophylline
D. Iron

15.You are attending to a man trapped in the driver's seat of a car. As firefighters attempt to extricate him from the vehicle, you notice that the patient's respiratory rate is 10 cpm. Pulse rate is 120 bpm, fast, and thready. Which of the following interventions is most appropriate?

A. Apply a cervical collar.
B. Give oxygen through a non-rebreather mask.
C. Defibrillate the patient.
D. Use the draw sheet method to extricate the patient.

16. You respond to a 32-year-old female with a bleeding scalp injury following a physical assault by unidentified men. What is the least likely feature you will find on examination?

A. Persistent bleeding
B. Traumatic brain injury
C. Bleeding into the skull
D. Decreased skull pressure

17. Which of the following is not a common sign of skull fracture?
   A. Absent carotid pulse
   B. Blood and CSF leakage from ear or nasal orifices
   C. Discoloration around the eyes
   D. Bruising around the mastoid process

18. All except which of the following are signs of Cushing reflex?
   A. Increased blood pressure
   B. Decreased pulse rate
   C. Irregular respiratory pattern
   D. Tachycardia

19. In the intensive care unit, you are briefed about a patient who is said to be unconscious and unresponsive, with dilated asymmetric pupils, decorticate posturing, and Cushing reflex. What might be the likely cause?
   A. Traumatic brain injury
   B. Open head injury
   C. Cerebral herniation
   D. Skull fracture

20. Spinal cord injury is commonly caused by which of the following?
   A. Acrobatics
   B. Motor vehicle collision
   C. Penetrating injury
   D. Fall from a height

21. Which of the following is false about the autonomic nervous system?
   A. The center is in the limbic system.
   B. It consists of the parasympathetic and sympathetic branches.
   C. The skeletal muscles do not receive impulses.
   D. Its function is involuntary.

22. You have the urge to urinate while driving home from work. As you drive, you almost hit a toddler, who strayed into the road. After a sudden swerve away from the child, you bring your car to a halt. Your heart is racing, you are sweating, and you no longer feel the urge to urinate. What is the most likely nervous system involved?
   A. Parasympathetic nervous system
   B. Sympathetic nervous system
   C. Central nervous system
   D. Both A and B

23. A victim of a motor vehicle collision is rushed to the ER. After a thorough assessment, it is determined that the victim's spinal cord was spared. Which of the following is not a protective skeletal component for the spinal cord?

A. Skull
B. Vertebrae
C. Pia mater
D. Intervertebral disc

24. Following a motorcycle crash, a patient was brought in with paralysis of the left lower limb and exaggerated reflex activities of upper limbs. A spinal injury is suspected. What is the least likely mechanism of injury?

A. Sudden lateral bending body
B. Spinal compression injury
C. Excessive extension, flexion or rotation
D. Fall on an outstretched arm

25. If conscious, the above patient may demonstrate all except which of the following signs and symptoms?

A. Tenderness in the area of injury
B. Weakness, numbness, and/or tingling sensation
C. Paralysis below the suspected level of injury
D. Paralysis above the suspected level of injury

26. After stabilizing the above patient, which of the following questions is not necessary for assessing responsiveness?

A. Do you have sudden neck or back pain?
B. Can you push your hand against mine?
C. Do you have any blurring of vision?
D. Do you feel my hand on your arm?

27. If the above patient is severely injured, your response as an EMT should include all except which of the following steps?

A. Placing the patient in a properly fitted cervical collar and minimizing spinal movement
B. Assessing the pulse, as well as the sensory and motor responses of the extremities
C. Performing airway control with in-line stabilization
D. Avoiding artificial ventilation with in-line stabilization

28. Another patient who was a passenger in the above motorcycle crash was later brought to the ER. He still has a helmet on. Under what conditions should you remove the helmet?

A. The helmet fits the patient with little or no head movement within the helmet.
B. There are no threatened airway or breathing difficulties.
C. You are unable to perform proper spinal immobilization.
D. There is a risk of causing more injury to the patient on removal of the helmet.

29. Which of the following is not a correct way of protecting a 7-year-old child after a suspected spinal injury?

A. Immobilize the child on a rigid board of appropriate size.
B. Use a pediatric collar device.
C. Manually tape a towel to the board to support the head and neck if the cervical immobilization device does not fit.
D. Pad the shoulders down to the heels to maintain neutral immobilization.

30. A 6-year-old male has severe facial lacerations after a head-on collision with an automobile. In your primary assessment of this patient, all except which of the following features are important to consider before triaging him as a high-priority patient?

A. Slow heart rate
B. Respiratory distress
C. Altered mental status
D. Hemorrhagia

31. Concerning secondary assessment of the above patient, which of the following is incorrect?

A. Skip the detailed examination if you realize the patient is unstable or a hospital is nearby.
B. For unstable patients, repeat assessment every 5 minutes.
C. Repeat assessment every 30 minutes for stable patients.
D. Inform the hospital about the patient's condition and treatment so far.

32. You are responding to a 4-year-old male with a foreign body in his left eye. Which of the following interventions is inappropriate?

A. Invert the left eye and remove the foreign body.
B. Patch the eye to reduce irritation.
C. Grasp the eyelid while telling the patient to look down.
D. Apply an applicator swab along the center of the upper eyelid.

33. You are responding to a male 36-year-old driver who sustained a facial trauma injury in a motor vehicle crash. Which of the following emergency responses is incorrect?

A. Thoroughly assess the facial tissue, oral cavity, teeth, and other facial organs.
B. If bleeding, regularly suction blood from the oral cavity.
C. Administer oxygen via positive pressure ventilation irrespective of respiratory condition.
D. Treat any teeth avulsion with saline gauze.

34. You are responding to a 12-year-old male with a bleeding nose following a fall on his face. Which of the following management protocols is unsuitable for this child?

A. Control all external bleeding.
B. Position him supine on the bed.
C. Examine him for nasal fractures and treat with cold compresses.
D. Never pack the internal nares with gauze.

35. A 65-year-old male slipped and fell with his occiput first on a staircase. He feels severe neck pain and headache. All except which of the following are basic interventions for this patient with a neck injury?

A. Assessing the airway and administering oxygen when necessary
B. Applying occlusion dressing for neck wounds
C. Immobilizing of the neck before transport
D. Attempting a direct laryngoscopy

36. You are attending to a 26-year-old female with profuse bleeding from a neck knife slit. Which of the following interventions is inappropriate in managing a severed neck blood vessel injury?

A. Apply as much pressure as possible to control bleeding.
B. Apply a regular bulky and occlusive dressing.
C. Quickly apply pressure on the carotid artery.
D. If the patient is not on oxygen therapy, commence it immediately and treat for shock.

37. Which of the following is the least likely form of eye injury?

A. Orbit injury
B. Lid injury
C. Globe injury
D. Impaled injury

38. You are called to the scene where a 17-year-old male has been having a seizure for over 10 minutes. Which of the following is an appropriate course of action?

A. Reassure onlookers and administer antiseizure medication.
B. Restrain the patient and remove harmful objects in the surroundings to prevent injury.
C. Insert a nasopharyngeal airway and commence positive pressure ventilation.
D. Commence high-concentration oxygen via a non-rebreather mask.

39. Concerning allergic reactions, which of the following is false?

A. They may resolve spontaneously without intervention.
B. Antigens are proteins that are formed in the body.
C. Symptoms may range from mild to life-threatening.
D. They are an intrinsic defense mechanism of the body.

40. Pathways through which the body may be exposed to allergens include all except which of the following?

A. Ingestion
B. Inhalation
C. Transformation
D. Absorption

41. Which of the following is correct concerning anaphylaxis?

A. It is typically an IgG-mediated reaction.
B. The reaction is always limited to one body system.
C. A sensitization stage is not necessary.
D. The response depends on individual sensitivity, rate, and dose of administration.

42. You are called to attend to a 15-year-old female who was sitting with her friends in a park. She reports she was stung by a wasp earlier and self-administered her prescribed epinephrine injection. Which of the following is not a side effect of epinephrine use?

A. Pallor
B. Dizziness
C. Bradycardia
D. Chest pain

43. Which of the following is false concerning anaphylactoid reactions?

A. They are clinically similar to anaphylaxis.
B. They do not involve IgE.
C. They require prior sensitization.
D. They occur via direct stimulation of mast cells or immune complexes.

44. Concerning epinephrine auto-injection, which of the following is false?
   A. The medication is in liquid form.
   B. The adult dose is 0.3 mg.
   C. The infant/child dose is 0.15 mg.
   D. The vial is usually packaged with a separate syringe and needle.

45. Which of the following is not a criterion for administering an epinephrine injection?
   A. Medication is prescribed for the patient by a physician.
   B. Medical direction authorizes use for the patient.
   C. It should be administered based on a patient's request, irrespective of prior prescription.
   D. The standing order of local protocol permits administration.

46. Concerning the management of allergic reactions, all except which of the following may be useful?
   A. Epinephrine
   B. Chlorpheniramine
   C. H1-receptor agonists
   D. Oxygen

47. All except which of the following are findings from the examination of a patient with an allergic reaction?
   A. Stridor, wheezing
   B. Cough, labored breathing
   C. Bradycardia, hypertension
   D. Pruritus, urticaria

48. All except which of the following are properties of carbon monoxide?
   A. Colorlessness
   B. Odorlessness
   C. Tastelessness
   D. Less affinity to hemoglobin than oxygen

49. You are called to the scene of a burning building where a 34-year-old female has just been rescued. On examination, she has increased pulse and respiratory rate. She also complains of headaches, weakness, vomiting, and blurred vision. All except which of the following are appropriate interventions?
   A. Commence high-flow oxygen.
   B. Administer antimotility agents.
   C. Remove the patient from continued exposure.
   D. Promptly notify the emergency department.

50. Which of the following is not necessary for the emergency management of poisoning?

A. Consult medical direction before administering medication.
B. Remove pills from the patient's mouth.
C. Collect all bottles, labels, and other packages of poisonous substances.
D. Collect a detailed history, including secondary assessment, before administering any intervention.

51. Activated charcoal is useful in the management of poisoning. Which of the following is an indication for administering this medication?

A. Ingestion of acids or alkalis
B. Vomiting
C. Altered mental status
D. Patient unable to swallow

52. You are the emergency responder to a 4-year-old female who was reported to have swallowed several tablets of Tylenol. You have received clearance from the medical direction to administer activated charcoal. Which of the following information is false?

A. The medication binds to certain poisons and prevents their absorption.
B. Side effects may include black stool and vomiting.
C. All brands of this medication are similar in efficacy.
D. The usual dose of this medication for infants/children is 12.5 to 25 g.

53. Serotonin syndrome can occur as a side effect of several medications. Which of the following combinations are not signs/symptoms of this syndrome?

A. Agitation, myoclonus, tremor
B. Incoordination, hyperreflexia, diaphoresis
C. Bradycardia, bradypnea, dry mouth
D. Hypertension, trismus, opisthotonus

54. A 16-year-old male was out at a party last night where inhalant recreational drugs were used. Which of these side effects will not be seen in the immediate period after the party?

A. Liver damage
B. Headache
C. Runny nose
D. Rashes around the nose and mouth

55. You are the emergency responder attending to a 21-year-old male who is disoriented, confused, and agitated. His roommate reports that he is a heavy drinker and suddenly stopped drinking alcohol three days ago. He has also been having visual hallucinations. On examination, the man's blood pressure is elevated. What is your most likely diagnosis?

A. Schizophrenia
B. Delirium tremens
C. Wernicke encephalopathy
D. Delirium

56. Which of the following is false concerning cocaine?

A. It is a strong CNS depressant.
B. It is a local anesthetic.
C. Abuse may result in acute myocardial infarction.
D. Routes of administration include oral, rectal and intranasal.

57. You are called to attend to an 18-year-old drug user who had a seizure. He is extremely diaphoretic on examination, with pupillary dilatation. He has a temperature of 37.7° C, a heart rate of 110 bpm, and a blood pressure of 144/92 mmHg. What is the most likely drug the young man abused?

A. Heroine
B. Ecstasy
C. Clonidine
D. Blue Nitro

58. Which of the following does not constitute a hazmat scene?

A. A diesel truck on fire
B. A leaking gas line in a household kitchen
C. A violent male in a public park
D. None of the above

59. Concerning hazmat incidents, which of the following is false?

A. Hazmat scenes are controlled by specialized teams.
B. EMS personnel are allowed to operate within hazmat scenes at any point.
C. Hazmat incidents require a specialized breathing apparatus.
D. EMS personnel who are not part of the hazmat team should operate only in the cold zone.

60. Concerning crime scenes, all except which of the following should be observed?

A. Under no circumstances should the crime scene be disturbed.
B. Scene security should always be controlled by a law enforcement agency.
C. The chain of evidence should be maintained as much as possible.
D. Assistance from law enforcement should be requested when in doubt.

61. Diseases of concern for pre-hospital personnel include all except which of the following?

A. Herpes simplex/syphilis
B. Meningitis/tuberculosis
C. Hepatitis B virus/human immunodeficiency virus
D. Rotavirus/hepatitis C virus

62. All except which of the following diseases are spread through air droplets?

A. Tuberculosis
B. Hepatitis C
C. Measles
D. Pertussis

63. Concerning PPEs, which of the following is false?

A. A surgical mask should be worn by care providers dealing with possible blood splatter.
B. A HEPA respirator should be used by care providers dealing with certain airborne diseases such as tuberculosis.
C. Gloves are optional, depending on the care provider's discretion.
D. Gowns are needed for large splash conditions.

64. Which of the following is a route of spread of communicable disease?

A. Indirect contact
B. Direct contact
C. Vector-borne
D. All of the above

65. Which of the following is not part of the EMS shift checklist for automated defibrillators?

A. Confirm that ventilators are working and all have clean tubing.
B. Check if the LED screen is okay.
C. Check if the batteries are okay.
D. Confirm that ECG paper is present.

66. Which of the following is true about sickle cell disease?

A. A person with the sickle cell trait has one sickle cell gene.
B. A person with sickle cell disease has red blood cells that become crescent shaped in the presence of hypocapnia.
C. Jaundice is a sign of sickle cell crisis only in children.
D. Dyspnea and chest pain are signs of sickle cell crisis.

67. Your team is called to a house party where a 23-year-old male has suddenly become breathless with facial puffiness and slurred speech. On arrival, you find the patient lying outside on the lawn with a crowd around him. His pulse is 122 bpm with a blood pressure of 84/56 mmHg. Respiratory rate is 12 cpm with wheezing, and oxygen saturation is 92%. A friend says the man has a nut allergy, and one of the cakes at the party had peanut butter in it. What is the most appropriate intervention?

A. Immediately try to pass an oropharyngeal airway to improve ventilation.
B. Immediately give supplemental oxygen.
C. Immediately administer IM epinephrine to the anterolateral aspect of the man's thigh.
D. Immediately administer IV steroids, preferably methylprednisolone, to counteract the anaphylactic reaction.

68. Which of the following is true about nitroglycerin?

A. It can be given sublingually as a tablet or a spray.
B. An EMT can give nitroglycerin to any patient with symptoms suggestive of angina.
C. Nitroglycerin decomposes when exposed to light or heat and must be kept in dark-colored, airtight plastic containers.
D. A side effect of nitroglycerin is hypertension.

69. Your unit arrives at a farmer's market where a 66-year-old female is having shortness of breath that started the previous day but suddenly got worse that afternoon. She has been coughing for a while now, and it affects her sleep. She recently noticed that she was easily fatigued from regular activities, like climbing the stairs. The woman tells you she is hypertensive but has reduced the dosage of her antihypertensives because they have become expensive. Her BP is 170/100 mmHg. Pulse rate is 100 bpm. Respiratory rate is 40 cpm. SpO2 is 90%. The woman's ankles are swollen, and her feet are cold. Which of the following steps is most appropriate?

A. Give the woman cough syrup for immediate relief, then move her to the vehicle for transportation.
B. Place the woman in a sitting position with her feet dangling and give supplemental oxygen to maintain saturation.
C. Immediately nebulize the woman to open up her airways before commencing CPAP.
D. Lay the woman in a supine position if possible; wrap her in a warm blanket and administer supplemental oxygen.

70. A 57-year-old female complains of chest pain for two hours. She also says her heartbeat is faster, it is more pronounced, and it "skips." Her breathing is labored. She says she is not hypertensive. While you are getting a history, the woman suddenly slumps over with no palpable pulse. What should you do?

A. Check the woman's vital signs and obtain a brief history before performing any other intervention.
B. Commence CPR immediately and give epinephrine if there is no improvement.
C. Commence CPR, then apply AED pads when available.
D. Lay the woman supine on the floor and commence supplemental oxygen.

71. Which of the following will not be present during septic shock?

A. Fever with cold extremities
B. Elevated blood pressure
C. Confusion
D. Fast heart rate

72. A 28-year-old male collapses after being told his pregnant wife just gave birth to quadruplets. His BP is 90/70 mmHg. His pulse is 74 bpm, and his respiratory rate is 16 cpm. The man's loss of consciousness is most likely due to which of the following?

A. Psychogenic shock
B. Dehydration
C. Heart attack
D. Neurogenic shock

73. You are administering CPR to a 35-year-old female who lost consciousness while using the elliptical machine at the gym. Which of the following are signs of effective CPR?

A. The chest rises and falls with ventilation.
B. Oxygen saturation is constant between 70% and 80%.
C. The abdomen swells with artificial respiration.
D. The heart rate becomes irregular.

74. You are attending to a 39-year-old diabetic who is bleeding actively from a laceration on his left foot after striking it against a stone. He does not feel much pain, but the bleeding, which has lasted about 30 minutes, concerns him. He has had an ulcer on his right foot for a month, which has not healed and is foul smelling. He also has occasional bouts of fever that usually abate after he takes some Tylenol. He is pale, his limbs are cold and his pulse is 118 bpm with a respiratory rate of 32 cpm. The bleeding is most likely due to which of the following?

A. Anemia as evidenced by pallor
B. Enzymes from a snakebite the man did not feel as a result of peripheral neuropathy
C. A side effect of frequent use of Tylenol
D. DIC that may have resulted from an infected foot ulcer

75. You are called to a Pilates class where the 50-year-old receptionist started complaining of difficulty in breathing and chest pain. Her pulse rate is 60 bpm, her blood pressure is 110/60mmHg, and her respiratory rate is 30 cpm with a SpO2 of 90%. The woman says that she has angina, and her prescribed nitroglycerin is in a bag in her locker. What do you do?

A. Lay the woman supine on the floor and start artificial respiration and chest compressions.
B. Keep the woman in a comfortable position, start her on supplemental O2, then administer her prescribed nitroglycerin.
C. Sit the woman on a chair and administer supplemental oxygen with a non-rebreather mask.
D. Immediately move the woman to your vehicle and transport her to a hospital.

76. Your team is called to a studio where a 51-year-old news presenter complains of squeezing pain on the left side of his chest that started while he was reading the 7 p.m. news. He says that he had a large meal and that the pain is most likely indigestion because he vomited before you arrived. Vomiting gave him a little relief. His blood pressure is 154/88 mmHg. His pulse rate is 90 bpm and his respiratory rate is 28 cpm. What is the most likely cause of this presentation?

A. A peptic ulcer aggravated by the big meal
B. A myocardial infarction
C. Pneumonia
D. Cardiogenic shock

77. You are called to the home of a 61-year-old female who suddenly woke up at night with chest pain, difficulty breathing, and a lack of energy. She is lying supine with a blood pressure of 90/68 mmHg, a pulse rate of 68 bpm, and a respiratory rate of 30 cpm. The woman's limbs are cool and pale. Her son, whom she lives with, says the woman has nitroglycerin she takes for her angina. Which of the following interventions will be beneficial?

A. Place the woman in a comfortable position, commence supplemental oxygen, and administer her prescribed nitroglycerin.
B. Place the woman in a sitting position, evaluate the need for oxygen, and administer supplemental oxygen if needed.
C. Lay the woman supine on the floor and commence high-quality CPR.
D. Place the woman in a supine position and commence supplemental oxygen; keep her warm and transport her immediately to a hospital.

78. A 60-year-old known hypertensive complains of sudden ripping pain in his chest and between his shoulder blades. He feels lightheaded and is sweating profusely with shortness of breath. His blood pressure is 182/92 mmHg in his right arm and 160/90 mmHg in his left arm. His pulse is 70 bpm. Which of the following steps is most appropriate?

A. Place the man in a comfortable position, maintain saturation with supplemental oxygen, and administer nitroglycerin.
B. Place the man in the Trendelenburg position and administer supplemental oxygen via a non-rebreather mask for adequate saturation.
C. Lay the man in a supine position in your vehicle, administer oxygen to maintain saturation, perform an ECG, and quickly transport him to the hospital.
D. Encourage the man to take his antihypertensives to normalize his blood pressure and ask him to see his cardiologist the following day.

79. Your team is at a marathon in July when you are notified of a spectator who collapsed while watching the race. When you get there, she is lying on the floor but has come to as bystanders sprinkle her with water. However, she is confused, her lips look cracked, and her skin is dry and hot. Her pulse rate is 108 bpm with a blood pressure of 148/90 mmHg and a rectal temperature of 40.5° C. You are unable to get a history, as nobody around seems to know the woman. What do you do?

A. Move the woman to the shade. Remove her clothes and place ice packs under her arms, on her neck, and in her groin to help reduce her body temperature.
B. Get the woman a bottle of water and encourage her to drink as much as possible to rehydrate.
C. Douse the woman with a bucket of water to cool her down, commence supplemental oxygen, then quickly transport her to a hospital.
D. Take off the woman's clothes and start cold-water immersion (CWI) immediately.

80. You are called to attend to a university football player who collapsed during team practice. You find him unconscious, with his teammates and coach around him. You take off the player's pads and clothes, then take a rectal temperature of 41° C. You prepare a tub to commence CWI. Which of the following is not beneficial to the process?

A. You can stop when he starts shivering or after 15 to 20 minutes of cooling.
B. Do not commence CWI until you have done a blood glucose check.
C. Move the water around the patient to increase the rate of cooling.
D. The rectal thermistor can remain in the rectum while the patient is being cooled down to allow for constant internal temperature monitoring.

81. Your unit is called to the scene of a road traffic accident on the interstate. You find an overturned car by the side of the road and a middle-aged male lying unconscious on the grass. Bystanders tell you that the driver was trying to avoid a fridge that fell off a moving truck. Which of the following are not important parts of assessing scene safety?

A. Scene assessment should be carried out continually throughout the call.
B. You should have an exit strategy in mind.
C. The call taker collecting valuable information from the 911 call is critical to scene safety.
D. You should use "why" questions to find out what the patient needs.

82. Your team is called to the scene of a motor vehicle accident where a 78-year-old female was struck by an SUV while crossing the street. You find her lying on the floor in a pool of blood, and you determine scene safety. The woman complains of severe pain in her left leg, which is bruised, lacerated, and swollen just below the knee and turned at an odd angle. The woman feels dizzy. Her pulse rate is 128 bpm and thready. Her blood pressure is 90/68 mmHg. Her hands and feet are cold. What is the most likely cause of this presentation?

A. Heart attack
B. Hypovolemia from blood loss
C. Third-space volume loss
D. Neurogenic shock

83. A 22-year-old male collapses on the front lawn of his house, prone with no palpable carotid pulse and no visible respiratory effort. You have already activated the emergency response system and called for a defibrillator. What is your next step?

A. Lay the man supine and wait for the AED.
B. Lay the man supine and give 30 chest compressions to two breaths while you wait for the AED.
C. Lay the man supine and give 10 to 12 rescue breaths per minute while you wait for the AED.
D. Quickly administer 1 mg of epinephrine via intraosseous access.

84. A 70-year-old male with chronic hypertension and diabetes has a productive cough, shortness of breath, mucopurulent sputum expectoration, fever, diaphoresis, reduced appetite, increased sleepiness, and lethargy. He had flu-like symptoms four days before his symptoms worsened. Pulse rate is 120 bpm, respiration is 26 breaths per minute, and auscultation reveals widespread rhonchi with reduced breath sounds in apical lung zones. What is the most likely prehospital diagnosis?

A. Pneumonia
B. Pulmonary embolism
C. Common cold
D. Pulmonary edema

85. All except which of the following are oxygen-delivery devices?

A. Venturi mask
B. Nasal cannula
C. Non-rebreather mask
D. Laryngeal mask

86. An 85-year-old female falls down a flight of stairs while trying to get to the bathroom at night. She is unconscious; her breathing is 8 breaths per minute, and her pulse is weak and thready. There is purplish discoloration under her eyes and bleeding from her ears. What is the most appropriate intervention?

A. Immediately lay the woman in the recovery position.
B. Commence suctioning vigorously without delay.
C. Perform a jaw thrust and start ventilation.
D. Perform chest compressions.

87. A 45-year-old male with detachable dentures gets into a fistfight with his neighbor. After receiving several blows to the jaw, he suddenly grabs his throat and starts making choking sounds, frantically moving his arms as his face turns purple. What is the most appropriate intervention?

A. Perform a jaw thrust while using a finger to sweep in the mouth.
B. Encourage the patient to cough.
C. Give abdominal thrusts.
D. Quickly give supplemental oxygen with a non-rebreather mask.

88. A 70-year-old farmer is found with altered consciousness and unresponsiveness. His neighbor reveals the farmer had gone to fumigate his farm four hours earlier. He has generalized seizures and is restless, agitated, and afebrile, with copious oral secretions. Pulse is 60 bpm, respiration is 10 breaths per minute, and blood pressure is 100/60 mmHg. What condition do you suspect?

A. Anaphylaxis
B. Seizure disorder
C. Organophosphate poisoning
D. Asthma

89. In what part of the lungs does gaseous exchange occur?

A. Trachea
B. Bronchi
C. Alveoli
D. Diaphragm

90. Which of the following patients has tachypnea?

A. A newborn with respiratory rate of 40 breaths per minute
B. A 16-year-old male with respiratory rate of 14 breaths per minute
C. A 2-year-old with respiratory rate of 36 breaths per minute
D. A 40-year-old with respiratory rate of 18 breaths per minute

91. Which of the following best defines tachypnea?
   A. Increased heart rate
   B. Difficulty breathing
   C. Increase in work of breathing
   D. Increased respiratory rate

92. The conducting zone of the respiratory system consists of all except which of the following?
   A. The trachea
   B. The bronchus
   C. The alveoli
   D. The terminal bronchiole

93. What part of the brain controls the rate of breathing?
   A. Pneumotaxic center
   B. Apneustic center
   C. Medullary respiratory center
   D. Cerebral cortex

94. A 40-year-old male presents with dyspnea of four days duration. What is his most likely condition?
   A. Difficulty breathing
   B. Fast breathing
   C. Shallow breathing
   D. None of the above

95. A 70-year-old male is dyspneic and agitated. He appears cyanosed. Which of the following best describes cyanosis?
   A. Bluish discoloration of the conjunctiva
   B. Warm, flushed, reddish skin discoloration
   C. Yellow discoloration of the skin and mucous membranes
   D. Bluish discoloration of the skin and mucous membranes

96. *Blue bloater* is a term used for patients with which of the following diseases?
   A. Atelectasis
   B. Chronic bronchitis
   C. Asthma
   D. Emphysema

97. A 60-year-old female with a history of COPD presents with cough and worsening shortness of breath. Which of the following features is suggestive of chronic bronchitis?

A. Thin appearance
B. Pursed-lip breathing
C. Bilateral lower limb swelling
D. Barrel chest

98. A 65-year-old male is dyspneic and has a chronic history of productive cough and recurrent chest infections. He appears cyanosed and is bloated with bilateral leg swelling. He is breathing with accessory muscles of respiration. On auscultation, rhonchi can be heard. SPO2 is 90%. What is the most likely prehospital diagnosis?

A. Chronic bronchitis
B. Emphysema
C. COPD
D. Asthma

99. A known asthmatic patient presents with dyspnea, altered consciousness, agitation, poor respiratory effort, and cyanosis. SaO2 is 88%, and the chest is silent on auscultation. These symptoms are a feature of which of the following?

A. A mild asthmatic attack
B. A moderate asthmatic attack
C. A severe asthmatic attack
D. A life-threatening asthma attack

100. A 44-year-old female suffered a blow to the head from assault. She is semi-conscious and responds to painful stimuli. She is drooling and has copious oral secretions. Snoring sounds can also be heard. What is the most appropriate intervention?

A. Give high-flow oxygen with a non-rebreather mask.
B. Suction with a rigid catheter.
C. Stabilize the spine and insert a nasopharyngeal.
D. Perform a jaw thrust, suction, and insert a nasopharyngeal airway.

101. What is the flow rate of a BVM?

A. 10 liters per minute
B. 15 liters per minute
C. 2 to 6 liters per minute
D. 12 liters per minute

102. BVM ventilation is contraindicated in which of the following conditions?

A. If there is a complete upper airway obstruction
B. If there is apnea
C. If there is hypoxic respiratory failure
D. If there is hypercapnic respiratory failure

103. A 30-year-old male was reported to be unconscious after a drinking spree with friends. He vomits while resuscitation is ongoing. You should do all except which of the following?

A. Move the tip of the suction catheter from side to side after suction is applied.
B. Insert the catheter into the oral cavity without suction.
C. Insert the suction catheter to the base of the tongue.
D. Suction for more than 30 seconds at a time.

104. A 20-year-old unconscious female rapidly produces frothy secretions while the EMT is artificially ventilating her. The EMT should do which of the following?

A. Suction for 15 seconds and ventilate for 2 seconds in an alternate manner.
B. Suction for 30 seconds and ventilate for 5 seconds in an alternate manner.
C. Suction for 10 minutes and ventilate for 4 minutes in an alternate manner.
D. Suction for 30 seconds and ventilate for 4 seconds in an alternate manner.

105. A 75-year-old male had a tracheotomy tube inserted for a malignant obstructing laryngeal tumor. His wife finds him unresponsive. On your arrival, he is markedly thin, febrile, and warm to touch, with minimal respiratory effort. His pulse is 40 bpm and blood pressure is 90/40 mmHg. You commence bag-to-stoma ventilations and notice air escaping through the man's nose and mouth with each breath. What should you do?

A. Reposition the jaw.
B. Reposition the man's fingers and mask.
C. Manually seal the man's mouth and nose.
D. Seal the man's stoma and ventilate from the mouth.

106. Flow-restricted oxygen-powered ventilation devices provide oxygen at which of the following peak rates?

A. 20 L/min
B. 30 L/min
C. 40 L/min
D. 50 L/min

107. You are called to a middle school where a 13-year-old male has been stung by a bee and is having difficulty breathing. He is wheezing. The bite site is red, itching, and swollen, and the boy's voice is now hoarse. His pulse is 110 bpm and weak, and the boy feels dizzy. His SpO2 is 90%. What do you do?

A. Administer IM epinephrine and supplemental oxygen, and transport the boy to the hospital.
B. Commence supplemental oxygen by BVM.
C. Remove the stinger and transport the boy to the hospital as soon as possible.
D. Move the boy to the vehicle and transport him to the hospital as quickly as possible.

108. Neighbors call your team to a home where a 15-year-old male has slit his wrists and is bleeding profusely. He is home alone with no adult around. He is conscious but weak, with agonal respiration. He refuses care from you. What is the most appropriate next step?

A. Hold off on treatment until you can get consent from a family member.
B. Counsel the patient on the severity of his condition and try to obtain consent as soon as possible.
C. Since the patient is a minor and consent cannot be obtained, you can go ahead and provide necessary medical services.
D. Immediately transport the patient to the hospital.

109. You and a colleague are resuscitating a 6-year-old female with cardiac arrest. The emergency response system has been activated, and a defibrillator is present. The child has no pulse and shows no respiratory effort. What is the most appropriate next step?

A. Commence defibrillation as soon as an AED is available.
B. Administer amiodarone via intraosseous access immediately.
C. Commence supplemental oxygen via intranasal cannula.
D. Call for an AED, but start CPR at 30 chest compressions to two slow breaths, attach the defibrillator when available, and assess.

110. You are giving chest compressions to a 2-week-old baby with no pulse and no respiratory activity. Which of the following is applicable?

A. Two-finger compressions at the xiphoid bone
B. Side-by-side thumb placement just below the nipple line
C. Hand positioned on the sternum
D. Both palms placed on either chest

111. Which of the following makes the pediatric airway more easily prone to blockage?

A. It is smaller and softer, and it has a longer, lower airway.
B. Infants have a proportionately larger tongue.
C. Infants have a flatter nose and face.
D. Infants' intercostal and accessory muscles are not well developed.

112. An 18-month-old male is apneic, and you are giving artificial ventilation with a BVM. What is the most correct statement pertaining to using BVM ventilation in a pediatric patient?

A. Pediatric patients' proportionately smaller tongues predispose them to blockages.
B. Hyperextending the neck helps open up the airway.
C. Pediatric patients' flatter and shorter noses may make creating a mask seal difficult.
D. Pediatric patients are not prone to gastric distention from positive pressure ventilation.

113. A 5-year-old male with a history of asthma and food allergies complains of a three-day history of cough, wheezing, and chest tightness. His mother says there are no clear triggers for his respiratory symptoms; however, he had mild symptoms of an upper respiratory tract infection. With the current episode, he has used his rescue inhaler more frequently without any relief. On examination, he has increased work of breathing, oxygen saturation is 90%, and respiration is 48 breaths per minute. Poor air entry to both lung bases is noted bilaterally, and there is wheezing in the upper lung zones. Which of the following is an appropriate intervention?

A. Give oxygen via a nasal cannula.
B. Administer nebulized albuterol.
C. Encourage steam inhalation.
D. Arrange for emergency transport.

114. An 18-month-old baby suffered a seizure and lapsed into unconsciousness. While resuscitation is ongoing, he gags, and secretions cover the airway. Which of the following catheters is most suitable for suctioning this child's airway?

A. Flexible suction catheter
B. Rigid suction catheter
C. Tip catheter
D. Suction bulb aspirator

115. Which of the following is the least likely indicator of child abuse?

A. Multiple bruises in various stages of healing
B. Injuries consistent with the mechanism described
C. Repeated calls to the same address
D. Child seems afraid to disclose how the injury occurred

116. Concerning sudden infant death syndrome, which of the following is incorrect?

A. The causes are many and not clearly understood.
B. EMT should try to resuscitate infants unless rigor mortis has set in.
C. Parents may feel emotionally distressed, remorseful, and guilty.
D. EMTs should attempt to educate the parents as much as possible while carrying out resuscitation.

117. You and your partner have been dispatched to a party where a 10-year-old male was rescued from a pool. He is responsive with normal vital signs, although he appears anxious. Which of the following is false concerning the management of near-drowning?

A. The possibility of trauma should be considered.
B. Hypothermia should be managed if present.
C. The boy does not need to be transported to the hospital if his vital signs are normal.
D. Alcohol ingestion should be considered.

118. You are attending to a 24-month-old child who is lethargic. Parents report that he has had diarrhea in the past 24 hours. On examination, his skin is pale and clammy with a delayed capillary refill. What is the most appropriate intervention?

A. Keep the boy warm.
B. Be prepared to artificially ventilate the boy.
C. Ensure a patent airway/oxygen.
D. All of the above.

119. Regarding the emergency management of an unresponsive poisoning patient, which of the following is false?

A. You should contact medical control.
B. You should rule out trauma.
C. You should consider the need to administer activated charcoal.
D. You should be prepared to artificially ventilate.

120. Your team arrives at a law firm to find an anxious 29-year-old lawyer who started feeling a tearing pain in his chest and back during his lunch break. The pain has been on and off for the past week. The man found he had trouble swallowing his food. He is also having difficulty breathing, has a wheeze, and says his voice has gotten hoarse. His blood pressure is 136/88 mmHg with a pulse of 110 bpm and respiratory rate of 20 cpm. The lawyer confides in you that he uses cocaine frequently and used some in the bathroom today before the pain started. What is the most likely cause of this presentation?

A. Anaphylactic reaction
B. Cardiogenic shock
C. Aortic aneurysm
D. Acute exacerbation of asthma

Test 2: Answers and Explanations

1. (C) Reassuring the families of the outcome of the patient
This method is inappropriate because grieving families should not be given false reassurances. Methods that can be used to help grieving families include therapeutic communication techniques, mindfulness of cultural and religious beliefs, answering questions when necessary, and silence.

2. (D) Regret
The five stages of grief are:
Denial – The person refuses to accept the diagnosis of death.
Anger – The person has accepted the diagnosis but is upset that it has to happen to them.
Bargaining – The patient resorts to making bargains to postpone the inevitability of death.
Depression – The patient realizes they are unable to postpone death and are sad.
Acceptance – The patient makes peace with the diagnosis.

3. (D) Meetings are supervised by a psychologist.
This statement is false because debriefings are peer-group meetings with no centralized leadership or supervision. This structure allows participants to talk freely and explore the emotions surrounding the incident.

4. (C) Mention only the patient's first name.
This is not a correct principle because radio waves are public and can be accessed by other parties. For this reason, the patient's name should not be mentioned.

5. (D) Using seat belts when driving
This is not a component of preassignment operations. Before an operation is assigned to a response team, the team prepares for the dispatch call by inspecting all equipment used for resuscitation; charging suction machines; checking the oxygen cylinders; inspecting the batteries for the AED; ensuring spare batteries are available; and ensuring that all supplies needed for wound care, splinting, and other materials for emergency care are available. Also, the functionality of the ambulance is assessed, ensuring that it is safe and ready for use.

6. (C) Using headlights
Option C is unlikely to reduce the chances of an ambulance crashing. Headlights are useful in notifying other drivers of the ambulance and providing illumination. Options A and B are incorrect because the unnecessary use of air horns and red lights increases the risk of accidents. Also, state laws control the use of air horns and red lights. Multiple ambulances and escort vehicles increase the risk of crashes at intersections.

7. (D) Slow down and stop if the light turns red.
This is the most appropriate response because it reduces the risk of vehicular crashes. Option A is incorrect because the use of air horns and red lights is controlled by local and state laws. Option B is incorrect because disobeying traffic signs can cause accidents. Option C is incorrect because maneuvering increases the risk of collision with other drivers and/or pedestrians.

8. (B) Unfamiliar routes
Multiple ambulances should be used only when the route to the patient or receiving facility is unfamiliar. The use of escorts and multiple ambulances is very dangerous. This protocol has a high risk of intersection crashes and collisions with motorists and pedestrians.

9. (B) Using sirens
To reduce the risk of collisions and intersection crashes of escorts and multiple ambulances, red lights, sirens and air horns should be avoided. Also, all vehicles must drive a safe distance from one another.

10. (D) It should be given as oral tablets.
This statement is false because albuterol is given as a nebulized solution. In adults and children, 0.083% is given over 15 minutes. It can be repeated to a maximum of three doses.

11. (C) Wheezing
Epinephrine is a sympathomimetic alpha and beta-adrenergic receptor agonist. It is used to treat bronchoconstriction, wheezing, and hypotension in patients with anaphylaxis.

12. (D) Blurred vision
Blurred vision is not a side effect of nitroglycerin. Side effects include postural hypotension, reflex hypertension, tachycardia, allergic reactions, diaphoresis, vomiting, and muscle twitching.

13. (D) Heparin
An EMT cannot administer heparin. Drugs that can be given by an EMT include oxygen, glucose, nebulized salbutamol/albuterol, aspirin, nitroglycerin, activated charcoal, epinephrine, and atropine/pralidoxime.

14. (D) Iron
Activated charcoal is an absorbent used for rapid absorption of most drugs (theophylline, digoxin, aspirin, acetaminophen, sedatives, and antidepressants). It is, however, not useful for absorbing alcohol, cyanide, caustics, iron, and lithium.

15. (B) Give oxygen through a non-rebreather mask.
This is the most appropriate intervention. This patient has respiratory failure either from hypovolemic or hemorrhagic shock; it is difficult to say which at the moment. Emergent care will include high-flow oxygen through a non-rebreather mask and rapid extrication. Option A is incorrect because although a cervical collar will reduce the risk of injury to the cervical spine, it cannot improve this patient's respiratory function. Option C is incorrect because the patient is not yet in cardiac arrest and therefore cannot be defibrillated. Moreover, oxygen must be given before an AED is used. Option D is incorrect because the draw sheet method is not useful in extracting a patient trapped in a vehicle.

16. (D) Decreased skull pressure
The least likely feature you will find on examination is decreased skull pressure. The scalp has good vasculature and, as such, may bleed more than expected. Depending on severity, bleeding may extend into the skull. This can cause increased pressure in the skull.

17. (A) Absent carotid pulse
An absent carotid arterial pulse is an unlikely finding in a skull fracture. An absent carotid pulse usually results from systemic conditions like aortic dissection.

18. (D) Tachycardia
Tachycardia is not a sign of Cushing reflex. Cushing reflex is a physiological response of the brain to increased levels of intracranial pressure. In Cushing reflex, there is increased arterial blood pressure triggered by the activation of the sympathetic nervous system from cerebral hypoxia. This stimulates baroreceptors in carotid bodies and causes the activation of the parasympathetic nervous system. The end result is bradycardia. There is also a classical irregular respiratory pattern due to impaired brain stem function caused by elevated intracranial pressure. Irregular respiratory pattern is a poor prognosis.

19. (C) Cerebral herniation
This patient has cerebral herniation. Typical signs are high blood pressure, loss of reflexes, and sometimes seizures. It is commonly caused by a head injury. In this condition, increased intracranial pressure forces the brain from its normal position down the skull.

20. (B) Motor vehicle collision
Motor vehicle collisions are the leading cause of spinal cord injury. The collisions cause a sudden, traumatic impact on the vertebrae, which dislocates, fractures, and crushes or compresses the spinal cord. Falling from a height is also a common cause of spinal cord injury, though mostly in the elderly. Its incidence is also greater than spinal cord injuries resulting from penetrating injuries like gunshots. Athletic activities like acrobatics or diving cause only a few spinal cord injuries.
21. (A) The center is in the limbic system.
This statement is false. The limbic system is the center for behavioral and emotional responses. The center of the autonomic nervous system is in the hypothalamus and conveys involuntary impulses to both cardiac and smooth muscles. The autonomic system controls involuntary actions of the body with innervations to smooth muscles and cardiac muscles. It is divided into the parasympathetic and sympathetic nervous systems.

22. (B) Sympathetic nervous system
The sympathetic nervous system is most likely involved, as it responds to fear, fright, and flight. Features include pupillary dilation, increased cardiovascular activity, decreased peristaltic movement, and increased secretions from the sweat glands.

23. (C) Pia mater
The bony framework supporting the spinal cord consists of the skull and the vertebral column or the spinal column, with the vertebrae bones and intervertebral discs as components. The pia mater and other parts of the meninges form a nonskeletal protective layer.

24. (D) Fall on an outstretched arm
The least likely mechanism of injury in this circumstance is a fall on an outstretched arm. That would most likely result in a humeral or ulnar fracture rather than a spinal cord injury. Compression injuries involving the spinal column and sudden excessive movement of the body—especially the back, on account of the impact of the crash—are mechanisms of spinal injury.

25. (D) Paralysis above the suspected level of injury
If conscious, the patient is unlikely to experience paralysis above the suspected level of injury. There is usually numbness or a tingling sensation, and in worse cases, loss of sensation below the suspected level of spinal cord injury. This is caused by loss of innervation from surrounding nerves and soft tissue inflammation.

26. (C) Do you have any blurring of vision?
This question is inappropriate for assessing responsiveness in this patient. A spinal cord injury is unlikely to affect vision. This can be explained more with cranial nerve two (optic nerve) injury or compression. Sensory and motor function and supply will be compromised to affected limbs due to the focus of spinal injury. Neck and back pain will help rule out any cervical injury. Examining the motor and sensory function of a patient is also important in assessing the severity of the injury.

27. (D) Avoiding artificial ventilation with in-line stabilization.
This step is not appropriate in this case. A severe spinal cord injury may affect respiratory function, especially if a cervical injury is involved with reduced air entry. In these patients, airway patency should always be ensured with artificial ventilation and oxygen therapy for respiratory support.

28. (C) You are unable to perform proper spinal immobilization.
Common reasons a helmet should be removed from victims include an inability to perform proper spinal immobilization, improperly fitting helmets, and an inability to assess or reassess airway and breathing.

29. (D) Pad the shoulders down to the heels to maintain neutral immobilization.
This is not a correct method of protecting a child after a suspected spinal injury. Padding of infants or children depends on the severity of spinal and associated injuries. It should be done only when necessary. Also, a poorly fitting cervical immobilization device will cause more harm to the child than good.

30. (A) Slow heart rate
This is not an important feature to consider before triaging the boy as a high-priority patient. A severe facial laceration can cause severe bleeding and hypovolemia. In worse cases, due to severe bleeding, the patient might go into shock and experience disorientation, altered mental status, respiratory distress, and loss of consciousness. Additionally, the patient may be exposed to eye injury (extrusion of the eyeball).

31. (C) Repeat assessment every 30 minutes for stable patients.
This statement is incorrect. For stable patients, it is recommended to repeat assessment every 15 minutes. Secondary assessment is completed when the patient is stable.

Depending on the severity and prognosis of the condition, skipping a detailed examination is necessary to ensure patients get adequate first-line management.

32. (B) Patch the eye to reduce irritation.
Patching the eye in an attempt to reduce irritation is both counterproductive and inappropriate, as this can create a humid environment for microorganisms.

33. (C) Administer oxygen via positive pressure ventilation irrespective of respiratory condition.
This response is incorrect. Oxygen should be given only if there is a need. The patency of the airway and oxygen saturation should be assessed to determine the patient's need.

34. (B) Position him supine on the bed.
This protocol is unsuitable. In the management of nasal bleeding, you should never put a patient in the supine position, as there may be bleeding into and obstruction of the airway. It is recommended that patients be positioned in a left lateral position to avoid aspiration pneumonitis.

35. (D) Attempting a direct laryngoscopy
This is not an appropriate intervention at this stage. A laryngoscopy is not basic care compared to other options, which are immediate and beneficial to controlling the patient's hemostatic balance. Immobilization of patients before transport is key. On further examination at an equipped facility, a laryngoscopy or bronchoscopy might be required.

36. (C) Quickly apply pressure on the carotid artery.
This intervention is inappropriate. You should apply digital pressure on the carotid artery only as a last resort to reduce blood loss. Digital pressure might compromise the blood supply to the brain and trigger brain tissue hypoxia and brain death.

37. (D) Impaled injury
This is the least likely form of eye injury. Most orbital injuries are orbital fractures following skull or facial trauma. Globe injury occurs when a blunt or penetrating injury disrupts the outer membrane of the eye. Its classification depends on the depth of penetration (in other words, whether the object penetrates the sclera or cornea).

38. (D) Commence high-concentration oxygen via a non-rebreather mask.
This is the most appropriate course of action. It is not practical to attempt to pass a nasopharyngeal airway tube in a patient with an ongoing seizure.

39. (B) Antigens are proteins that are formed in the body.
This statement is false. Antigens that elicit allergic reactions gain access into the body from an external source and are not formed within the body.

40. (C) Transformation
Option C is false. The pathways through which allergens enter the body include injection, inhalation, absorption, and inhalation.

41. (D) The response depends on individual sensitivity, rate, and dose of administration.
This statement is correct. Usually, anaphylaxis is mediated by IgE and includes a prior sensitization stage. Symptoms may include one or more systems.

42. (C) Bradycardia
Bradycardia, a slower heart rate, is not a side effect of epinephrine use. Epinephrine mimics a sympathetic nervous discharge; hence, a patient may experience an increased heart rate. Other possible side effects include excitability or anxiousness, headaches, nausea and vomiting.

43. (C) They require prior sensitization.
This statement is false. An anaphylactoid reaction is clinically similar to anaphylaxis, except that it is not an IgE-mediated reaction and requires no prior sensitization.

44. (D) The vial is usually packaged with a separate syringe and needle.
This statement is false. An epinephrine auto-injector is a single unit consisting of a needle and syringe system and so does not require a separate needle and syringe. An adult auto-injector contains 0.3 mg of epinephrine per vial, while a pediatric auto-injector holds 0.15 mg.

45. (C) It should be administered based on a patient's request, irrespective of prior prescription.
This is not a criterion for administering epinephrine. The decision to administer epinephrine should be based on local protocol and medical direction and not depending on a patient's request, especially if other criteria have not been met.

46. (C) H1-receptor agonists
Histamine is released when mast cells are degraded. It stimulates histamine receptors, which stimulate allergic reactions. H1-receptor agonists will worsen allergic reactions. On the contrary, antagonists, such as chlorpheniramine, are useful, as they bind to these histamine receptors, thereby preventing receptor stimulation. Depending on the severity of an allergic reaction (anaphylaxis), supplemental oxygen and epinephrine injection may come in handy.

47. (C) Bradycardia, hypertension
An increase in heart rate and a decrease in blood pressure (hypotension) are more in keeping with findings in an allergic reaction.

48. (D) Less affinity to hemoglobin than oxygen
These are not properties of carbon monoxide. Carbon monoxide has a higher affinity to hemoglobin than oxygen; this complex is known as carboxyhemoglobin.

49. (B) Administer antimotility agents.
This is not an appropriate intervention. Preventing further exposure to carbon monoxide while optimizing oxygen delivery are the most important aspects of managing poisoning. Antimotility agents have no role in this management.

50. (D) Collect a detailed history, including secondary assessment, before administering any intervention.
This is not necessary for the emergency management of poisoning. In the management of victims of poisoning and other emergencies, the intervention must be undertaken as soon as possible. Time spent carrying out a secondary assessment and collecting a detailed history may be costly for the patient. Remember to call medical direction for clearance before administering any medication. Also, retrieve all indicators of the likely poison ingested and take them along to the hospital.

51. (B) Vomiting
An indication for administering activated charcoal is vomiting. The dose may be repeated once if the patient vomits after taking the medication.

52. (C) All brands of this medication are similar in efficacy.
This statement is false. The binding capacity of activated charcoal differs among brands; hence, medical direction should be consulted about the brand to use.

53. (C) Bradycardia, bradypnea, dry mouth
These are not signs of serotonin syndrome. Features include an increased heart rate and respiratory rate.

54. (A) Liver damage
Liver damage is a long-term effect of inhalant drug abuse and is usually not seen immediately.

55. (B) Delirium tremens
Delirium tremens is a life-threatening condition from alcohol withdrawal. Symptoms commonly occur within 72 hours after the last drink but may arise later.

56. (A) It is a strong CNS depressant.
This is false concerning cocaine. The effects of cocaine are caused by its CNS stimulant activities. The drug accelerates certain body functions.

57. (B) Ecstasy
The symptoms listed are characteristic of amphetamine abuse. Blue Nitro and heroin are CNS depressants and will cause hypotension, bradycardia, and bradypnea, among other symptoms.

58. (C) A violent male in a public park
Although the safety of a scene should be assessed before proceeding to offer services, a violent male in a public park is not considered a hazmat scene.

59. (B) EMS personnel are allowed to operate within hazmat scenes at any point.
This is false. EMS personnel should restrict their operations to the cold zone until the hazmat team has certified an area as safe.

60. (A) Under no circumstances should the crime scene be disturbed.
This is false. Crime scenes may be disturbed when it is required for medical care; however, a minimal disturbance should be maintained.

61. (D) Rotavirus/hepatitis C virus
While the other listed diseases pose a significant source of infection to emergency responders, rotavirus and hepatitis C cause a comparatively milder illness.

62. (B) Hepatitis C
The mode of transmission of hepatitis C is through contact with infected blood, not air droplets.

63. (C) Gloves are optional, depending on the care provider's discretion.
This is false. Gloves should be worn before every assignment to reduce the risk of exposure to infectious agents. It is necessary to change your pair of gloves before attending to a new patient and to wash your hands before and after every EMS activity.

64. (D) All of the above
Communicable diseases may be spread from direct contact with infected patients, from vectors, or through contact with inanimate objects around infected persons.

65. (A) Confirm that ventilators are working and all have clean tubing.
Ventilators are not part of the EMS shift checklist for AEDs.

66. (D) Dyspnea and chest pain are signs of sickle cell crisis.
This statement is true. Dyspnea and chest pain can be seen in sickle cell crises as a condition called acute chest syndrome.

67. (C) Immediately administer IM epinephrine to the anterolateral aspect of the patient's thigh.
Epinephrine should be given immediately in anaphylaxis. It is the drug of choice, as it causes bronchodilation and vasoconstriction. Based on the history provided by the friend and the patient's vital signs, this patient is most likely in anaphylactic shock. Supplemental oxygen is important but should not be the first step, and IV steroids will not have any immediate effect.

68. (A) It can be given sublingually as a tablet or a spray.
This statement is true. Nitroglycerin comes in both tablets and sprays, which are administered sublingually. It should not be kept in plastic bottles, as it is volatile and readily absorbed by most plastics, reducing its efficacy. Hypotension is one of its side effects. An EMT can administer nitroglycerin if it is already prescribed, it is available, and the patient's systolic pressure is above 100 mmHg.

69. (A) Give the woman cough syrup for immediate relief, then move her to the vehicle for transportation.
This step is most appropriate. The patient's symptoms and history are in keeping with congestive heart failure. Sitting her up will be beneficial to improve oxygen saturation. The cough and shortness of breath are most likely due to fluid buildup in her lungs, and laying the patient down will worsen this. Nebulization will not improve saturation, as the patient's airways are not constricted.

70. (C) Commence CPR, then apply AED pads when available.
Immediate defibrillation is the first line of action for cardiac arrest. However, CPR should not be delayed while you wait for the AED.

71. (B) Elevated blood pressure
Elevated blood pressure is not seen in septic shock. In septic shock, hypotension (not hypertension) is seen due to widespread vasodilation caused by inflammatory mediators. Confusion, fever, and an increased heart rate are all features of septic shock.

72. (A) Psychogenic shock
The man's loss of consciousness is most likely due to psychogenic shock. Psychogenic shock is a sudden reaction of the nervous system to fear, bad news, etc., producing temporary, generalized vasodilation.

73. (A) The chest rises and falls with ventilation.
Good chest rise is an indicator that the lungs are being appropriately ventilated by CPR. Oxygen saturation and heart rate should also improve.

74. (D) DIC that may have resulted from an infected foot ulcer
The bleeding is most likely due to an untreated diabetic foot ulcer. The ulcer has most likely progressed to become septic, which eventually activated the patient's coagulation pathway, depleting his clotting factors.

75. (B) Keep the woman in a comfortable position, start her on supplemental O2, then administer her prescribed nitroglycerin.
Placing the patient in a position of comfort helps her anxiety; administering supplemental oxygen ensures adequate saturation. Since the patient has been prescribed nitroglycerin and her systolic pressure is above 100 mmHg, the medication can legally be administered by an EMT.

76. (B) A myocardial infarction
An MI usually presents with chest pain similar to that of an ulcer. With the patient's elevated blood pressure, however, it is unlikely to be a peptic ulcer, pneumonia, or cardiogenic shock.

77. (D) Place the woman in a supine position and commence supplemental oxygen; keep her warm and transport her immediately to a hospital.
The patient is most likely in cardiogenic shock. Laying her in a supine position will reduce the workload on the heart. Nitroglycerin causes vasodilation, which will further lower the woman's blood pressure. Supplemental oxygen will improve saturation.

78. (C) Lay the man in a supine position in your vehicle, administer oxygen to maintain saturation, perform an ECG, and quickly transport him to the hospital.
These steps are most appropriate to take. The disparity in blood pressures in the man's arms should raise a high suspicion for acute aortic dissection or an aneurysm. The definitive treatment for this is surgical, so the man should immediately be transported to a hospital with cardiothoracic capabilities.

79. (D) Take off the woman's clothes and start cold-water immersion (CWI) immediately.
Cold-water immersion will cool the patient fastest and is the gold standard. In heatstroke, timely, rapid cooling is critical. As an adequate history cannot be obtained from this patient, it is best to treat this case as such. Oral intake is ill-advised.

80. (B) Do not commence CWI until you have done a blood glucose check.
This step is not beneficial to the process. A blood glucose check should not delay CWI. All three other options add to the effective cooling-down of the patient. Move the patient to the hospital quickly for rehydration.

81. (D) You should use "why" questions to find out what the patient needs.
This is not an important part of assessing scene safety. "Why" questions tend to put people on the defensive instead of calming them down. All the other options are important to scene assessment and safety.

82. (B) Hypovolemia from blood loss
Hypovolemia is the most likely cause of this presentation, as the patient has lost a lot of blood from what seems to be a left leg fracture. This explains the hypotension, tachycardia, dizziness, and cold limbs. A heart attack usually presents with chest pain.

83. (B) Lay the patient supine and give 30 chest compressions to two breaths while you wait for the AED.
According to AHA guidelines, if a patient collapses with no pulse or breathing, CPR is the next step.

84. (A) Pneumonia
The most likely hospital diagnosis is pneumonia. Pulmonary embolism presents with chest pain and fast breathing of sudden onset with a history of associated risk factors. In pulmonary edema, orthopnea and crackles are heard in the base of the lungs. The common cold is not associated with mucopurulent sputum expectoration.

85. (D) Laryngeal mask
A laryngeal mask is not an oxygen-delivery delivery. It is a supraglottic airway device that is used during a pending respiratory arrest when endotracheal intubation cannot be achieved. The Venturi mask, nasal cannula, and non-rebreather mask help in the delivery of oxygen to patients in cases of respiratory distress.

86. (C) Perform a jaw thrust and start ventilation.
This is the most appropriate intervention. as the scenario suggests a basilar skull fracture from trauma. Facial fractures, cervical spine injury, intracranial hemorrhage, cranial nerve injury. and vascular injury can complicate basilar skull fractures. Performing a jaw thrust will open the airway and prevent worsening of a cervical spine injury. Starting ventilation will improve oxygen saturation. Great care should be taken while immobilizing the patient and securing the airway to avoid worsening the cervical spine/cranial nerve injury. Placing the patient in a recovery position is not beneficial. There is no history of copious secretions, so suction and CPR are not indicated.

87. (C) Give abdominal thrusts.
This is the most appropriate intervention, as dislodged dentures are the most likely cause of asphyxia in this patient. Give abdominal thrusts or Heimlich maneuvers to help relieve airway obstruction. The patient is not unconscious, so a jaw thrust and finger sweep are not indicated. You can encourage a patient to cough if he has a strong cough reflex to relieve his airway; however, this is not the case in this scenario, as this patient is exhibiting choking signs and is unable to cough. Relieving airway obstruction should be prioritized over giving supplemental oxygen because the patient is still conscious.

88. (C) Organophosphate poisoning
The patient's symptoms of altered consciousness, seizures, restlessness, agitation, and history of fumigating his farm point to organophosphate poisoning. Other symptoms of organophosphate poisoning include diarrhea, lacrimation, emesis, miosis, sweating, and confusion. Most pesticides are made of organophosphates, and poisoning can occur in farmers through inhalation and skin absorption. This can also occur among industrial workers who do not use appropriate safety gear.

89. (C) Alveoli
The gaseous exchange takes place in the alveoli. The alveoli, alveolar duct, and respiratory bronchioles make up the respiratory zone of the respiratory system and are the site for gaseous exchange. Conducting airways have no alveoli and do not play a role in gas exchange. The trachea and bronchi make up part of the conducting airway of the respiratory tract. The diaphragm is a muscular structure that separates the thoracic cavity from the abdominal cavity; contraction of the diaphragm aids respiration.

90. (C) A 2-year-old with respiratory rate of 36 breaths per minute
The average respiratory rate of a 2-year-old is about 20 to 30 breaths per minute. Values above this are considered tachypnea. All other patients in the question have respiratory rates within the normal range.

91. (D) Increased respiratory rate
In tachypnea, breathing is fast and shallow, and this increases the respiratory rate. Increased heart rate is tachycardia. An increase in work of breathing is a feature of respiratory distress. There is use of accessory muscles of respiration. It may also be associated with tachypnea. Difficulty in breathing refers to dyspnea (a common feature of respiratory distress), respiratory failure, or respiratory arrest.

92. (C) The alveoli
The alveoli make up part of the respiratory zone of the respiratory system. The conducting zone has no alveoli and does not play a part in gaseous exchange. The conducting zone of the respiratory tract includes the nostrils, pharynx, larynx, trachea, bronchi, and bronchioles.

93. (B) Apneustic center
The apneustic center, located in the lower pons, controls the rate of breathing. Lesions in this area of the brain cause pathological respiratory rhythm with increased apnea frequency. The pneumatic center in the upper pons regulates volume and rate of respiration through its inhibitory effect on the apneustic center. The medullary respiratory center controls inspiration, and the cerebral cortex controls activities such as breath-holding while talking, coughing, or vomiting.

94. (A) Difficulty breathing
The man most likely is suffering from dyspnea, meaning difficult or labored breathing. It is an uncomfortable feeling of awareness of breathing and is sometimes referred to as air hunger. Fast or rapid breathing is referred to as tachypnea. Breathing may be shallow in certain disease conditions, such as asthma, pneumonia, hyperventilation, anxiety, and pulmonary edema.

95. (D) Bluish discoloration of the skin and mucous membrane
This best describes cyanosis, as it is caused by hypoxia and results in blue discoloration of the skin and mucous membrane.

96. (B) Chronic bronchitis
Chronic bronchitis causes inflammation of the lining of the bronchus and copious mucus production in the respiratory tract. This impairs the conduction of gaseous exchange in the lungs, causing hypoxia and cyanosis. The increased strain on the heart leads to right-sided heart failure and edema, hence the term *blue bloater*. In atelectasis, chronic bronchitis, and severe and life-threatening asthma, cyanosis may occur; however, edema is uncommon.

97. (C) Bilateral lower limb swelling
This is a common feature of chronic bronchitis and occurs as a result of right-sided heart failure. A rail-thin appearance, barrel chest deformity, and pursed-lip breathing are symptoms of emphysema.

98. (A) Chronic bronchitis
The history of dyspnea, productive cough, cyanosis, and bloating with reduced SaO2 is suggestive of chronic bronchitis. Asthma presents with airway hyperresponsiveness and wheezing. In emphysema, edema is uncommon, and COPD is a spectrum of chronic airway diseases.

99. (D) A life-threatening asthma attack
These symptoms are a feature of life-threatening asthma. During asthma attacks, airway limitation can be severe and airflow insufficient. Affected patients may quickly progress from rhonchi to silent breathing. This is an ominous sign and usually precedes respiratory failure. A silent chest is not a feature of mild, moderate, or severe asthmatic attack.

100. (D) Perform a jaw thrust, suction, and insert a nasopharyngeal airway.
In this patient, you should perform a jaw thrust to avoid worsening any cervical spine injury. Suction the airway to clear copious secretions and insert a nasopharyngeal airway to prevent the tongue from blocking the airway. This will also prevent the patient from gagging during insertion of the oropharyngeal airway.

101. (B) 15 liters per minute
The BVM has an oxygen flow rate of 15 liters per minute.

102. (A) If there is a complete upper airway obstruction
BVM ventilation is contraindicated in a complete upper airway obstruction. The main goal in this case is to relieve obstruction and secure the airway. The BVM can be used in apnea, hypoxic respiratory failure, and hypercapnic respiratory failure to ventilate patients.

103. (D) Suction for more than 30 seconds at a time.
During resuscitation, suctioning should be limited to 15 seconds in adults. The suction catheter should be inserted into the oral cavity without suction. The catheter must be inserted to the base of the tongue or as far as you can see. While suctioning, move the tip of the catheter from side to side after suction is applied.

104. (A) Suction for 15 seconds and ventilate for two seconds in an alternate manner.
This is the correct sequence of suctioning and giving ventilations in an adult. Suction times for children and infants are fewer so that adequate ventilation can be given.

105. (C) Manually seal the man's mouth and nose.
Creating a seal over the man's mouth and nose when ventilating through a stoma can help prevent air leaks and improve ventilation. Sealing the stoma and ventilating through the mouth and nose can be useful if insufficient ventilation is from an obstruction in the stoma. Jaw and finger repositioning are not helpful to prevent air leaks in this case.

106. (C) 40 L/min
Flow-restricted oxygen-powered ventilation devices supply 100% oxygen at a flow rate of 40 liters per minute. They help improve oxygen saturation in patients with hypoxia.

107. (A) Administer IM epinephrine and supplemental oxygen, and transport the boy to the hospital.
The boy's symptoms and presentation are indicative of anaphylactic shock. A small percentage of people experience a severe allergic reaction to a bee sting. IM epinephrine is the gold standard and should be administered every 5 to 10 minutes until the patient improves.

108. (C) Since the patient is a minor and consent cannot be obtained, you can go ahead and provide necessary medical services.
Under the emergency exception rule, you can presume consent and proceed with treatment and transport as long as the following four conditions are met:

- The child has an emergent condition.
- The legal guardian of the child is unable to give consent or is unavailable.
- Transportation and treatment cannot be delayed until consent is given.
- The EMT professional gives the treatment that can reduce the child's life-threatening condition.

109. (D) Call for an AED, but start CPR at 30 chest compressions to two slow breaths, attach the defibrillator when available, and assess.
Once cardiac arrest is confirmed, it is best to commence CPR immediately while waiting for the AED. This reduces delay and improves prognosis.

110. (B) Side-by-side thumb placement just below the nipple line
Side-by-side thumb placement is the preferred and most effective for chest compressions in neonates.

111. (B) Infants have a proportionately larger tongue.
Infants have a proportionately larger tongue, and this blocks the airway and requires more careful positioning to maintain patency. The upper airway is smaller, shorter, and softer. This also makes the airway prone to block easily. A flatter nose and face make it more difficult to create a mask seal when providing ventilation on pediatric patients. The intercostal and accessory muscles are not well developed; hence, they depend more on the diaphragm for breathing.

112. (C) Pediatric patients' flatter and shorter noses may make creating a mask seal difficult.
It may be more difficult to create a good mask seal when providing ventilation due to a flatter nose and face, such as those seen in a pediatric patient. The tongue is proportionately larger in these patients and may cause occlusion of the airway. The neck needs to be placed in a neutral position, not hyperextended, to keep the airway open. Gastric distention from positive pressure ventilation is common in pediatric patients.

113. (B) Administer nebulized albuterol
The goal of asthma exacerbation treatment is to relieve exacerbation and return patients to their best lung function. Inhaled bronchodilators (beta-2 agonists and anticholinergics) are the mainstay of asthma treatment. The use of a nebulizer is preferred for younger children because of difficulties coordinating MDIs and spacers. Oxygen therapy is indicated because of hypoxia; however, a bronchodilator should be given as the first line to reverse airway limitation. Arrange for transport while nebulizing the patient. Steam inhalation will not help alleviate the symptoms.

114. (B) Rigid suction catheter
A hard or rigid suction catheter (also known as a tonsil sucker, tonsil tip, or Yankauer catheter) is most suitable for suctioning the mouth and oropharynx of children. It is also used to suction the mouth and oropharynx of an unresponsive patient. The rigid catheter should be inserted only as far as you can see. When rigid catheters are used for infants and children, caution should be taken not to touch the back of the airway, as this can trigger laryngeal spasms.

115. (B) Injuries consistent with the mechanism described
Of all the scenarios listed, this is the least likely indication of child abuse. Child abuse is a serious harm to children, and EMTs must know how to recognize this problem.

116. (D) EMTs should attempt to educate the parents as much as possible while carrying out resuscitation.
Any comments that may suggest blame or increase the feeling of guilt in the parents should be avoided. Parents should be counseled later in a more appropriate setting.

117. (C) The boy does not need to be transported to the hospital if his vital signs are normal.
This statement is false. Secondary drowning syndrome, which is deterioration after normal breathing, can occur minutes to hours after a near-drowning event; therefore all near-drowning victims should be transported to the hospital.

118. (D) All of the above.
All of the measures listed are appropriate interventions to take. Additionally, infants and children in shock need to be transported rapidly to the hospital, with secondary examination completed en route if time permits.

119. (C) You should consider the need to administer activated charcoal.
Activated charcoal should be considered only in the emergency management of a responsive patient.

120. (C) Aortic aneurysm
The most likely cause of this presentation is an aortic aneurysm. Such aneurysms usually present with tearing chest pain or pain between the shoulder blades. The risk is usually higher with increasing age, but in young people, it is associated with drug use. If a thoracic aneurysm grows large enough, it can compress surrounding structures.

Test 3: Questions

1. You have been dispatched to the residence of a 6-year-old female who is having a seizure. Her parents report that she has had previous episodes of seizures and is on medication. Which of the following is false concerning this patient's management?
   A. Position the girl on her side if there is no possibility of cervical spine trauma.
   B. Have suction ready.
   C. The patient will not require transportation once the seizure is aborted.
   D. None of the above.

2. Concerning the management of croup, which of the following is false?
   A. The Wesley score is used to grade severity.
   B. A Wesley score of 9 indicates the child is at risk of respiratory failure.
   C. Reduction of stridor is a good sign in children previously demonstrating signs of severe obstruction.
   D. None of the above.

3. Which of the following is true about epiglottitis?
   A. It occurs exclusively in children.
   B. The causal organism is a virus.
   C. Incidence has been reduced with the advent of a vaccine.
   D. Children are usually afebrile with drooling, hoarseness, and stridor.

4. Concerning the pediatric airway, which of the following is false?
   A. The tongue and jaw are proportional.
   B. Infants are obligate nose breathers.
   C. The pediatric airway is more anterior than in adults.
   D. Children can compensate well following respiratory compromise.

5. You have just assessed a 14-month-old baby who is said to have breathing problems. Which of the following is not a sign of mild airway obstruction in this patient?
   A. Good air exchange
   B. Coughing forcefully
   C. High-pitched snoring noise while inhaling
   D. None of the above

6. General assessment of a child can be obtained from the child's overall appearance. Which of the following should an EMT assess?

A. Mental status
B. Color
C. Interaction with parents
D. All of the above

7. The pediatric assessment triangle (PAT) is used to examine infants and toddlers. Which of the following is correct concerning PAT?

A. Appearance – mental status, muscle tone
B. Work of breathing – ventilatory rate, effort
C. Circulation – skin signs, color
D. All of the above

8. Concerning the assessment of children with traumatic injuries, which of the following is incorrect?

A. Blunt injury is most common.
B. It may result from child abuse.
C. Signs of trauma always appear early in the injury.
D. The pattern of injury is usually different from adults.

9. Your unit is called to an apartment building where a 4-year-old male has been coughing for about two weeks. He has a fever, which is on and off. His mother has been giving him cough syrup and Tylenol with only temporary improvement. The boy developed a high fever this morning, with vomiting and fast breathing. His mother says he suddenly started speaking illogically as she was preparing to take him to the hospital. The boy's pulse rate is 156 bpm. Respiratory rate is 50 cpm and temperature is 39° C with cold limbs. What is the most appropriate intervention?

A. Lay the boy supine, commence supplemental oxygen, and give IV fluids if authorized while preparing him for transport.
B. Lay the boy in a modified Trendelenburg position and administer oxygen with BVM.
C. Give IM epinephrine and move the boy to the vehicle for immediate transportation.
D. Commence immediate intubation for effective oxygen saturation.

10. A 12-year-old female suddenly slumps on the sidelines during a soccer match while trying to help an injured teammate with a leg fracture from a bad tackle. Her coach says the girl held the injured limb and suddenly collapsed. Her pulse rate is 100 bpm with a respiratory rate of 24 cpm . She has cold, clammy skin. As you are obtaining the girl's vitals, she wakes up. What is the most likely cause of her presentation?

A. Anaphylaxis
B. Dehydration
C. Cardiac arrest
D. Psychogenic shock

11. Which of the following is least likely to be a cause of pallor in a 12-year-old male?

A. Upper GI bleeding
B. Sepsis
C. Anaphylaxis
D. HbSC

12. You are performing CPR for a 6-month-old female in cardiac arrest. You attach an AED, and it shows ventricular fibrillation. You shock once, deliver CPR for two minutes, and reassess. The AED indicates no shockable rhythm. What is the next step?

A. Give one more shock with the AED to make sure.
B. Continue CPR for two more minutes.
C. Give about 12 to 20 rescue breaths in a minute.
D. Give IV or IO Amiodarone.

13. A 2-year-old female presents with a two-week history of paroxysmal cough and fever, which has gradually become worse. She has prolonged coughing spells that expectorate thick mucoid sputum. The girl is restless and takes deep breaths after each coughing bout. Her mother looks anxious. The girl's respiration is 36 breaths per minute, and pulse is 120 bpm. For this patient, what is your most likely prehospital diagnosis?

A. Croup
B. Epiglottitis
C. Pertussis
D. Pneumonia

14. For the 2-year-old patient above, what is an appropriate intervention?

A. Separate the girl from her anxious mother.
B. Give the girl oral acetaminophen.
C. Suction to the clear airway of mucoid sputum.
D. Administer humidified supplemental oxygen after taking universal precautions.

15. A 1-year-old boy was found unconscious after consuming pills from an aspirin bottle. He has no respiratory effort and his pulse is weak. Which of the following is an appropriate intervention?

A. Give rapid infusion of N-acetyl cysteine.
B. Give oxygen via a nasal cannula.
C. Commence BVM ventilation.
D. Identify the number of pills the boy swallowed in order to calculate the quantity of antidote.

16. A 4-year-old male with cystic fibrosis recently has had acute worsening of his symptoms and heavy mucus production. What is the most appropriate management?

A. Help the patient into a comfortable position and suction.
B. Insert an oropharyngeal airway.
C. Give an oral mucolytic.
D. Arrange for transport.

17. Which of the following is not the purpose of a prehospital care report?

A. Billing
B. Continuity of care
C. Evaluation of care
D. Chain of custody

18. You are attending to a 34-year-old female with syncope from heart failure. She has refused to go to the ER. After assessing her competence and educating the patient on the consequences of her refusal, you hand her the patient refusal form to sign. This patient refuses to sign. Which of the following interventions is most appropriate?

A. Sign in the patient's place.
B. Inform the dispatch officer.
C. Have a family member sign in the patient's place.
D. Document the patient's refusal to sign.

19. With the above patient, you are expected to fill out the primary care report before leaving. You will fill out all except which of the following pieces of information?

A. Patient assessment
B. Emergency care that should have been given
C. Patient education on available alternatives of care
D. Patient education on counseling and psychotherapy services

20. You are filling out a patient care report when you notice an error you made in the patient's address. Which of the following methods is most appropriate in erasing the error?

A. Begin with a new sheet.
B. Cover up the error with Wite-Out.
C. Sign on top the error.
D. Draw a single horizontal line through the error.

21. Which of the following is correct about a mobile receiver/transmitter?

A. It is mounted on vehicles.
B. It rebroadcasts transmissions at high frequency.
C. It can be used at a considerable distance from the vehicle.
D. It has a limited range.

22. You are attending to a 25-year-old African American female with anaphylaxis from a drug reaction. You are about to receive medical direction from a physician via a phone call. You are required to provide what information to the physician?

A. The patient's age
B. The patient's ethnicity
C. The patient's name
D. The patient's clinical state

23. Concerning the above patient, the doctor gives a prescription of epinephrine, 0.3 mg IM, stat. Which of the following is appropriate for clarifying the dose of this drug?

A. Write the order on paper.
B. Ask the physician to send the order as a text.
C. Repeat the order back to the physician.
D. Have your partner write the order on paper.

24. You have just transported a 35-year-old female with shortness of breath and chest tightness to the receiving center. As you prepare to hand the patient off to the emergency nurse, you receive a call for a motor vehicle accident two blocks away from where you are. You and your partner decide to answer the call. Which of the following is being described?

A. Duty of care
B. Negligence
C. Abandonment
D. Malpractice

25. All except which of the following are situations in which an EMT can give health information to a third party without the patient's consent?

A. Continuity of care
B. Billing
C. Subpoena to testify
D. Education of family members

26. Your team is the first to respond to a terrorist attack at a shopping mall. Which of the following roles is assigned to your team?

A. Transport
B. Triaging
C. Incident command
D. Extrication

27. As the incident commander responsible for attending to victims of a mass shootout, which of the following interventions must you perform first?

A. Stage the victims.
B. Call for backup.
C. Assess the safety of the location.
D. Ask those who can stand to do so.

28. You are triaging a group of victims involved in a motor vehicle accident. Which of the following should be done first?

A. Ask patients who can stand to do so.
B. Locate the dead patients.
C. Locate the bleeding patients.
D. Count the number of patients.

29. You are triaging a female with an open fracture of the thigh. She has altered consciousness but is oriented in place. Respiratory rate is 35 cpm. Her radial pulse is fast and thready. This patient will be triaged as which of the following?

A. Red
B. Black
C. Yellow
D. Green

30. You are triaging a male with burns to the arms, thighs, and legs. Respiratory rate is 25 cpm, radial pulse is present, and capillary refill is less than two seconds. The man can obey simple commands. This patient will be triaged as which of the following?

A. Red
B. Black
C. Yellow
D. Green

31. You are triaging a male with an open head injury. There is no respiratory effort, even after repositioning the airway. The radial pulse is absent. This patient will be triaged as which of the following?

A. Red
B. Black
C. Yellow
D. Green

32. Which of the following may be a potential source of threat to an EMT at a rescue incident?

A. Downed electrical lines
B. Explosions
C. Fire
D. All of the above

33. Which of these items may not be essential to an emergency responder to a hazmat scene?

A. Binoculars
B. Emergency response guidebook
C. Placards on buildings and trucks
D. None of the above

34. Regarding the Glasgow Coma Scale, which of the following is true?

A. The score ranges between 0 and 15.
B. It can be used in persons of all ages.
C. It assesses only functions of the central nervous system.
D. Scores are given based on verbal and motor responses and eye-opening.

35. Concerning motor response on the Glasgow Coma Scale, which of the following is incorrect?

A. No response – 1
B. Localizes pain – 4
C. Obeys command – 6
D. Extends to pain – 2

36. You are the first responder to a 63-year-old semi-conscious male. He opens his eyes to pain and has confused speech. He is also able to withdraw from painful stimuli. What is this patient's score on the Glasgow Coma Scale?

A. 11
B. 12
C. 10
D. 9

37. A 59-year-old male with type 2 diabetes is sitting by a sidewalk. He complains of weakness and is diaphoretic. On examination, his pulse is rapid and weak. Which of the following is a contraindication to administering oral glucose?

A. Gag reflex is absent.
B. It is unknown if he has taken his medication today.
C. Medical direction is absent.
D. His age.

38. All except which of the following can precipitate hypoglycemia?

A. Chronic alcoholism
B. Sepsis
C. Beta-agonists
D. Fasting

39. Which of the following is false concerning insulin?

A. It decreases serum glucose.
B. It increases glucose metabolism.
C. Secretion from beta cells is stimulated by high blood glucose.
D. None of the above.

40. You are called to attend to a 57-year-old male patient with poorly controlled diabetes. His daughter tells you he complained of abdominal pain earlier and had several episodes of vomiting. On examination, he has fruity-smelling breath with deep, rapid respiration. His pulse is rapid. Which of the following interventions is inappropriate?

A. Calling for ALS
B. Monitoring vital signs
C. Monitoring and maintaining the airway
D. Administering oral glucose

41. You have been dispatched to the residence of a 45-year-old female, where her distraught daughter informs you that the woman has become unresponsive. Which of the following will not be necessary in assessing this patient?

A. Length of coma
B. Onset of coma
C. History of drug abuse
D. None of the above

42. A change in a patient's mental status indicates an underlying neurological pathology. Which of the following may be responsible for this presentation?

A. Head trauma
B. Stroke
C. Sepsis
D. All of the above

43. A behavioral emergency is a situation in which people exhibit behavior that is abnormal and intolerable to them, their family, or their community. All except which of the following factors may alter a person's behavior?

A. Excessive temperature changes
B. Low blood sugar
C. Psychogenic factors
D. None of the above

44. Studies have shown several conditions that may be linked to an increased risk of suicide. Which of the following individuals has the lowest risk of suicide?

A. A 43-year-old alcoholic living by himself
B. A 39-year-old divorcee who has been out of a job
C. A 36-year-old female who is married and has flexible work hours
D. An 18-year-old college student who is depressed

45. The EMS has been notified of a 19-year-old student in a dormitory who is reported to be violent and tearing his room apart. Which of the following should be considered during a primary assessment?

A. Are there suicidal tendencies?
B. Has any intervention been given?
C. How does the patient feel?
D. All of the above

46. You and your partner have been dispatched to a neighborhood following a call that a resident has been yelling and breaking plates. His neighbors are unsure if any injury has been inflicted. Which of the following is false concerning emergency management?

A. You should assess the scene and ensure personal safety before approaching the patient.
B. The patient may be left alone for no more than 10 minutes.
C. You should ensure the patient stays calm as much as possible.
D. There may be a need to restrain the patient.

47. You and your partner are part of the rescue team of a 25-year-old female involved in a road traffic accident with several fatalities. She is unable to remember her name, phone number, or Social Security number; however, she can recall where she was heading and what she was going to do. What is the most likely diagnosis?

A. Somatization disorder
B. Depersonalization
C. Conversion disorder
D. Amnesic psychogenic dissociative disorder

48. You have been dispatched to a local bar where the owner reports that a guest who had been heavily drinking is now intoxicated and yelling. Which of the following points is not important to note when assessing this patient?

A. Potential for violent behavior
B. Possible inaccurate medical history
C. Possible abnormal responses to physical problems
D. None of the above

49. Dystonia can be a reaction to medications. It can present as muscle spasms involving the tongue, neck, and jaw. Which of the following medications is used to treat this condition?

A. Compazine
B. Cogentin
C. Thorazine
D. Haldol

50. In some cases, an emotionally disturbed person may resist medical treatment. Which of the following is false?

A. On no occasion should force be applied.
B. To provide care against a person's will, there must be a reasonable belief that a patient is at risk of self-harm or harm to others.
C. A patient may be transported without consent in some situations.
D. None of the above.

51. All except which of the following will protect an EMT against false accusations?

A. Documentation of abnormal behavior exhibited by a patient
B. Presence of a same-sex attendant
C. Having a witness in attendance during transportation
D. Avoiding reasonable force when indicated

52. You are the emergency responder to a 35-year-old female who is bleeding through her vagina. All except which of the following may be done?

A. Packing the vaginal canal with a dressing
B. Maintaining body temperature
C. Giving supplemental oxygen if necessary
D. Keeping the patient in a supine or left lateral position if in shock

53. A 19-year-old female is in severe abdominal pain and appears anxious. She complains of feeling faint and has seen small amounts of blood on her underwear. Her last menstrual period was two months ago. On examination, her heart rate is 108 bpm with a blood pressure of 100/70. What is your likely diagnosis?

A. Pelvic inflammatory disease
B. Ectopic pregnancy
C. Menorrhagia
D. Abnormal uterine bleeding

54. All except which of the following should be considered when obtaining a history from a gynecological patient?

A. Making a diagnosis of pregnancy
B. Having a trusted friend or family member present
C. Getting a full menstrual and sexual history
D. Obtaining a history of contraceptive use

55. A 55-year-old female complains of hot flashes, sudden mood changes, and irregular menses. Which of the following is the most likely explanation for this?

A. Depression
B. Early menopause
C. Menopause
D. Premature ovarian failure

56. You are attending to a 17-year-old female who complains of severe pain and cramping. During your assessment, you notice no abnormal vital signs, and her past medical history is insignificant. She is on the second day of her menstrual cycle. What is the most likely diagnosis?

A. Menorrhagia
B. Dysmenorrhea
C. Ectopic pregnancy
D. Premenstrual syndrome

57. You are dispatched to the home of a 19-year-old female whose last menstrual period was two weeks ago. She complains of severe and constant lower abdominal pain, nausea, and vomiting. She also admits to having fever, chills, and foul vaginal discharge. She has multiple sexual partners and has unprotected sexual intercourse. What is your most likely diagnosis?

A. Ectopic pregnancy
B. Pelvic inflammatory disease
C. Peptic ulcer disease
D. Premenstrual syndrome

58. Which of the following is not a sexually transmitted disease?

A. Syphilis
B. Chlamydia
C. Hepatitis A
D. Phthirus pubis

59. An 18-year-old known asthmatic becomes very emotional on receiving news of her mother's passing; she is sobbing hysterically. She is taking rapid and deep breaths. Her relatives have been unable to calm her. The woman is tachypneic with a respiratory rate of 30 cpm. On auscultation, vesicular breath sounds are heard. The woman also complains of numbness in her hands and feet, blurred vision, headaches, and dizziness. The woman most likely has which of the following?

A. Acute respiratory distress syndrome
B. Hyperventilation syndrome
C. Acute asthmatic attack
D. Acute coronary syndrome

60. Modifiable risk factors for pulmonary embolism include all except which of the following?

A. Combined oral contraceptive pills
B. Obesity
C. Cigarette smoking
D. Blood-clotting disorders

61. A 30-year-old obese male with a history of diabetes, high blood pressure, and ulcerative colitis, as well as a recent history of surgical repair of a femoral neck fracture, experiences sudden onset of dyspnea, cough, chest pain, and shortness of breath. His SPO2 readings are 90%, and crepitations are heard in lower lung zones on auscultation. Which of the following is the most likely prehospital diagnosis?

A. Acute pulmonary embolism
B. Pneumonia
C. Angina pectoris
D. Myocardial infarction

62. A child was rescued from a burning building. He is unconscious and having ineffective respirations. His mother is anxious and hysterical. What is the most important intervention?

A. Secure the child's airway and establish adequate ventilation.
B. Provide emergency transport.
C. Take a detailed history of the child.
D. Reassure the child's parents.

63. A 70-year-old obese female with hypertension complains of shortness of breath. Her symptoms started four days ago and have gotten worse. She is dyspneic with flaring of nostrils. She had similar symptoms a year ago when she had an acute COPD exacerbation. The woman has no history of fever, cough, or wheezing. She has bilateral pitting pedal edema, blood pressure 100/60 mmHg, 98 bpm, SPO2 92%. On auscultation, there are lung crackles and reduced air entry bilaterally. What is the most likely prehospital diagnosis for this patient?

A. Pulmonary embolism
B. Pulmonary edema
C. Acute respiratory distress syndrome
D. Bronchiolitis

64. While administering positive pressure ventilation to a patient, you notice massive gastric distention. What should you do?

A. Insert a nasopharyngeal airway.
B. Reposition the patient's head.
C. Create a tight mask seal.
D. Insert a nasogastric suction tube.

65. Which of the following is/are contraindications to insertion of a nasopharyngeal tube?

A. Sinusitis
B. Recent nasal surgery
C. Esophageal varices
D. All of the above

66. An asthmatic requires medication to open the bronchioles and reverse airflow limitation. What are these medications called?

A. Mucolytics
B. Bronchodilators
C. Corticosteroids
D. Mast stabilizers

67. Which of the following adjuncts is less likely to stimulate vomiting in a responsive patient at risk of airway obstruction?

A. Nasopharyngeal airway
B. Oropharyngeal airway
C. Endotracheal tube
D. Nasogastric tube

68. A 17-year-old unconscious female requires an oropharyngeal airway to prevent her tongue from blocking the airway. What is the most appropriate method for determining the proper size of the oropharyngeal airway?

A. Measure from the corner of the patient's lips to the ramus of the mandible.
B. Measure from the tip of the patient's nose to the tragus of the ear.
C. Measure from the sternal angle to the tip of the patient's nose.
D. Measure from the sternal angle to the outer corner of the patient's mouth.

69. A 30-year-old male is in a car crash. Upon your arrival at the scene, he is unconscious and apneic. What method should be used to open up the airway to assist ventilations?

A. Head-tilt/chin-lift
B. Jaw thrust
C. Log-rolling technique
D. Chin sweep lift

70. Infant breathing mainly depends on which of the following?

A. The nose
B. The mouth
C. The diaphragm
D. None of the above

71. Which of the following best describes a respiratory drive where the respiratory cycle is regulated by oxygen chemoreceptors and not carbon dioxide chemoreceptors?

A. Hypoxic drive
B. Hypercapnic drive
C. Hyperventilation syndrome
D. Central apnea

72. What are some common causes of airway compromise?

A. The tongue
B. Foreign body
C. Allergic reaction
D. All of the above

73. An EMT has successfully restored adequate spontaneous ventilation in a 35-year-old patient with respiratory distress using a flow-restricted oxygen-powered ventilation device. The patient's SPO2 in room air is 98%. He wants to discontinue oxygen usage. Which of the following steps is correct?

A. Remove the device from the patient, turn off the valve, and remove all pressure from the regulator.
B. Turn off the valve, remove the device from the patient, and remove all pressure regulators.
C. Remove all pressure regulators, turn off the valve, and remove the device from the patient.
D. None of the above.

74. A 40-year-old male complains of sudden onset of dyspnea, acute chest pain, and shortness of breath after a blunt injury to the chest. He is peripherally cyanosed, SPO2 90%, blood pressure 90/60 mmHg, pulse 120 bpm. The trachea deviates to the left, breath sounds are absent in the lower left lung zones, and there are hyperresonant percussion notes. What is your most likely prehospital diagnosis?

A. Tension pneumothorax
B. Myocardial infarction
C. Acute chest syndrome
D. Flail chest syndrome

75. A 45-year-old diabetic on combined oral contraceptives is being managed for a suspected pulmonary embolism. This is a result of occlusion of the blood supply to which of the following?

A. Pulmonary artery
B. Pulmonary vein
C. Inferior vena cava
D. Superior vena cava

76. An elderly diabetic is lethargic and dyspneic with deep, fast respirations. The patient is markedly dehydrated and has fruity breath. SaO2 is 90%. What is the appropriate intervention?

A. Provide supplemental oxygen.
B. Encourage the patient to breathe into a paper bag.
C. Commence chest compressions.
D. Determine the patient's random blood glucose.

77. A 24-year-old male is dyspneic, agitated, in respiratory distress with nasal flaring, and having subcostal and intercostal muscle retractions. He had a mucopurulent cough and upper respiratory tract symptoms a week before his symptoms worsened. His skin appears dusky. Pulse oximeter readings are 70 bpm and SPO2 is 90%. What should you do?

A. Administer oxygen with a Venturi mask.
B. Give blow-by humidified oxygen.
C. Administer oxygen with the nasal cannula at 4 L/min.
D. Give supplemental oxygen with a non-rebreather mask.

78. A 70-year-old hypertensive with COPD is dyspneic, complains of cough and frothy sputum, and has difficulty breathing on lying down. On your arrival, he is lying in bed, blood pressure 200/140 mmHg, pulse rate 90 bpm. There is bilateral pedal edema, and crackles are heard in the lung zones on auscultation. Which of the following is an appropriate intervention?

A. Assist the patient into an upright position with his feet dangling for comfort.
B. Place the patient in the lateral recovery position.
C. Administer a rescue inhaler.
D. Give blow-by humidified oxygen.

79. A 19-year-old male with impending respiratory failure requires continuous positive airway pressure. Which of the following is an indication of continuous positive airway pressure?

A. Cardiogenic pulmonary edema
B. Hypoxemic respiratory failure
C. Obstructive sleep apnea
D. All of the above

80. Concerning abnormal breath sounds, which of the following is true?

A. Stridor is a high-pitched harsh sound heard on inspiration.
B. Stridor is a high-pitched harsh sound heard on expiration.
C. Stridor is a sign of lower airway obstruction.
D. Stridor is heard on inspiration and expiration.

81. You are required to ventilate a patient with a tracheostomy tube. Which of the following is the most appropriate description of a tracheostomy?

A. A permanent artificial opening in the trachea
B. An artificial opening in the larynx
C. An artificial opening in the pleural cavity
D. None of the above

82. A 25-year-old female who is pale and weak with yellowing of the eyes complains of severe waist pain that began two days ago and has progressively worsened. Her blood pressure is 100/72 mmHg. Pulse rate is 100 bpm, and respiratory rate is 30 cpm. She tells you she has sickle cell disease. Which of the following is least likely to be this woman's genotype?

A. HbSS
B. HbSC
C. HbAC
D. HbSB+

83. Which of the following is a protocol in administering high-quality CPR?

A. Performing CPR in the prone position if you cannot get the patient in a supine position
B. Performing chest compressions at a rate of 20 to 30 per minute
C. Administering simultaneous compressions and ventilations
D. Performing chest compressions and ventilations at a ratio of 30:2

84. You are called to the home of a 40-year-old male who developed a bruise on his right knee about three weeks ago, to which he applied some penicillin ointment. He has progressively deteriorated with fever, weakness, and nausea. His wife says he is acting confused. You find the man lying on a couch with a swollen right knee. He is disoriented but conscious and has cold, clammy skin. His pulse rate is 112 bpm, blood pressure is 92/60 mmHg, and respiratory rate is 30 cpm. What is the most likely cause of this presentation?

A. Dehydration
B. Sepsis
C. Hypovolemic shock
D. Food poisoning

85. You and another EMT arrive at the scene of a mugging where a woman has been stabbed on both forearms and is actively bleeding. Her husband says the assailants tried to stab her in the neck, but she shielded herself. The woman is shaken but conscious and seated on the floor. Her husband is applying direct pressure to her wounds. What should you do?

A. Take over applying pressure, elevate the woman's hands, wrap a pressure dressing around the wound, and transport her to a hospital.
B. Apply a tourniquet distal to lacerations, commence the woman on oxygen, and transport her to a hospital.
C. Commence the woman on oxygen and transport her to a hospital.
D. Apply pressure on the woman's brachial artery, commence supplemental oxygen, and transport her to the nearest hospital.

86. A 43-year-old female complains of piercing chest pain radiating to her left arm and back. She has had trouble swallowing since yesterday, and her breathing is fast and wheezy. Her respiratory rate is 28 cpm with a blood pressure of 130/70 mmHg. Her pulse rate is 106 bpm. Which of the following is the most likely cause of this presentation?

A. Anaphylaxis
B. Aortic aneurysm
C. Congestive heart failure
D. Acute severe asthma

87. A 23-year-old male complains of itching and has breathing difficulties after taking his roommate's antibiotic capsules for his cough. When you arrive, he has a red rash all over his torso and is itching, with watery eyes and a runny nose. He has shortness of breath with a wheeze, respiratory rate of 32 cpm, and SPo2 of 90%. His blood pressure is 84/56 mmHg, and his pulse rate is 140 bpm. The man is not aware that he has any allergies. What is the most appropriate next step?

A. Give an antihistamine syrup immediately and commence supplemental oxygen.
B. Give oral prednisolone to stop the anaphylactic reaction.
C. Administer IV or IO epinephrine immediately and give supplemental oxygen.
D. Administer IV hydrocortisone immediately and commence oxygen.

88. A 68-year-old hypertensive and diabetic male presents supine with severe left-sided chest pain, which began suddenly during a game of tennis. He says he also experienced the same pain, which radiated to his jaw, while he was having his morning jog. His blood pressure is 138/74 mmHg, pulse rate is 90 bpm, and SPo2 is 92%. His respiratory rate is 26 cpm. Which of the following will the man most benefit from?

A. Place him in a comfortable position, administer supplemental oxygen, and carry out an ECG.
B. Administer nitroglycerin and transfer the man to a hospital immediately.
C. Administer an analgesic, carry out an ECG, then transport the man to a hospital.
D. Give the man his antihypertensive, commence supplemental oxygen, and transport him to the hospital immediately.

89. Your unit is called to an office complex where a 40-year-old female suddenly collapsed. You find her lying on the floor unconscious with cold, clammy skin and blood pressure of 86/54 mmHg. She has a weak pulse with a pulse rate of 120 bpm. Her respiratory rate is 32 cpm with a wheeze and crackles on auscultation. Her SPo2 is 88%. What is the most appropriate next step?

A. Lay the woman supine, commence CPR, and transport her to the hospital immediately.
B. Lay the woman supine, administer oxygen via CPAP, and transport her to a hospital immediately.
C. Sit the woman on a chair and administer supplemental oxygen via a non-rebreather mask.
D. Administer IV epinephrine, commence supplemental oxygen, and transport the woman to the hospital.

90. Nitroglycerin is most likely indicated in which of the following conditions?

A. Chest pain with a blood pressure of 88/56 mmHg with a doctor's prescription of nitroglycerin
B. Shortness of breath with SPo2 of 90%
C. Chest pain with a blood pressure of 132/70 mmHg with a doctor's prescription of nitroglycerin
D. Abdominal pain with vomiting and diarrhea

91. Which of the following is not part of the five steps of using an AED?

A. Power on the AED.
B. Attach electrode pads to the patient's skin.
C. Analyze the rhythm.
D. Administer a shock while your partner is administering rescue breaths.

92. A 30-year-old construction worker fell from a ladder at the first-floor level onto the pavement below. You meet him lying supine, in severe pain, with his right arm grotesquely positioned. There is no blood, and the man is conscious. His blood pressure is 96/66 mmHg, and his pulse rate is 56 cpm with deep breathing. His SPo2 is 92%. His skin is warm and flushed. What is the most likely cause of this presentation?

A. Hypovolemia
B. Cardiogenic shock
C. Acute coronary syndrome
D. Neurogenic shock

93. You are called to the home of a 76-year-old male who suddenly complained of stabbing pain in his chest and between his shoulder blades. This pain also radiates to his right jaw. Which of the following is a differential diagnosis for this pain?

A. Peptic ulcer
B. Pneumonia
C. Aortic aneurysm
D. Myocardial infarction

94. A 44-year-old known hypertensive male suddenly develops chest pain while taking a hike with his friends. You find him sitting on the ground, clutching his chest. He is weak and breathless. His blood pressure is 146/80 mmHg, and his pulse rate is 28 cpm. The man tells you that he forgot to take his antihypertensives that morning and shows you his medications—amlodipine, lisinopril, and nitroglycerin. What should you do?

A. Administer supplemental oxygen and the man's prescribed nitroglycerin, perform an ECG, and transport him to a hospital.
B. Administer the man's antihypertensives and commence supplemental oxygen before transporting him to a hospital.
C. Commence rescue breathing with a BVM and apply AED electrodes.
D. Move the man to a hospital immediately.

95. You are called to a shopping mall where you find a 21-year-old who suddenly became breathless. You find him sitting on a bench, dyspneic with a pulse rate of 118 bpm. He is pale and weak with cold limbs. He tells you his genotype is HbSB and that he has gotten worse and worse since he went on a vegetarian diet a month ago. He regularly takes folic acid and hydroxyurea. What should you do?

A. Lay the man in the Trendelenburg position, commence supplemental oxygen, and transport him to a hospital.
B. Lay the man in a supine position, place him on supplemental oxygen, keep him warm, and transport him to a hospital.
C. Set up IV access and hydrate the man with IV fluids.
D. Commence intranasal oxygen and apply AED pads.

96. You are using an AED on a patient with no pulse and agonal breathing. You have administered one shock, and the AED has analyzed. It still indicates shockable rhythm. What should be your next step?

A. Start CPR immediately.
B. Administer another shock to a maximum of three shocks if VF persists.
C. Intubate to ensure effective saturation.
D. Immediately transport the man to a hospital.

97. You are attending to a 47-year-old male with suspected ventricular fibrillation. You have placed the AED pads on his chest in the ambulance, and you are ready to transport him to a hospital. Which of the following is applicable?

A. Analyze the man's heart rhythm while in transport and, if necessary, stop the vehicle to deliver a shock.
B. Stop the vehicle if heart rhythm analysis is necessary and deliver a shock if needed.
C. Do not analyze the man's heart rhythm until you get to the hospital.
D. Stop the vehicle, analyze the man's heart rhythm, and deliver the shock while he is being transported.

98. You are attending to a 41-year-old male who is complaining of a headache of a day's duration. His blood pressure is 198/98 mmHg with a bounding pulse rate of 102 bpm. He is not hypertensive but says he has had two episodes of elevated blood pressure, for which he was given anxiolytics. Which of the following is the most likely cause of this presentation?

A. Hypertensive urgency
B. Cardiogenic shock
C. Ventricular fibrillation
D. Hypoglycemia

99. You are called to attend a delivery truck driver who collapsed in front of his house. When you arrive, he is lying supine on the front lawn, conscious but lethargic. He tells you he has been passing watery stools since the previous day. His blood pressure is 100/72 mmHg with a pulse rate of 98 bpm, shortness of breath, and dry mouth. What is the most likely cause of this presentation?

A. Hypertension
B. Hypothyroidism
C. Cardiogenic shock
D. Dehydration

100. You are called to a restaurant where a 29-year-old has suddenly developed a swollen throat and tongue with difficulty breathing and itching. He tells you he is allergic to most seafood and that he informed his waiter. What is the most likely cause of this presentation?

A. Acute asthma
B. Respiratory tract infection
C. Anaphylaxis
D. Urticaria

101. Which of the following should be the first course of action for a patient in anaphylactic shock?

A. Supplemental oxygen
B. Steroids
C. Epinephrine
D. Antihistamines

102. Concerning management for impaled objects to the cheeks, which of the following is incorrect?

A. Assess the stability of the patient and pack each side of the wound.
B. Assess for airway obstruction by an object.
C. Remove the impaled object in the direction of entry.
D. Remove the object from the opposite direction and pack both sides of the wound.

103. Which mechanism of injury does not explain what may happen to a patient with an open chest injury after an encounter with armed robbers?

A. Lung collapse from air trapped within the pleural space
B. Hemothorax as a result of vascular damage
C. Audible sucking sound due to air being pulled in through the hole on the chest
D. Decreased heart rate with warm and moist skin

104. Which of the following is unlikely after a closed chest injury?

A. Costochondritis
B. Pneumothorax
C. Tension pneumothorax
D. Flail segments

105. In a patient with tension pneumothorax, which of the following is correct?

A. Decreased or absent breath sounds on both sides
B. Increased breath sounds on both sides
C. Increased breath sounds on the affected side
D. Decreased or absent breath sounds on the affected side

106. In assessing a patient with chest injuries, you should do all except which of the following?

A. Assess the mechanism of injury to determine if it is a closed or open chest injury.
B. Ensure airway patency with a chin tilt irrespective of suspected cervical injury.
C. Take into account body substance isolation.
D. Ensure an in-line manual stabilization is taken.

107. In the emergency management of a patient with a chest injury, which of the following is contraindicated?

A. Providing oxygen at 15 L/min
B. Removing any impaled object from the patient
C. Occluding any soft tissue injury
D. Completely immobilizing the patient

108. Chest injuries with immediate life-threatening impacts include all except which of the following?

A. Flail segment
B. Open chest injury
C. Massive hemorrhage
D. Tracheal deviation

109. In trauma assessment of a victim of an abdominal injury, which of the following steps is incorrect?

A. Transport the patient from the scene immediately, irrespective of safety.
B. Size up the scene, assessing for safety.
C. Establish the mechanism of injury.
D. Assess for other victims at the scene of the injury.

110. In the assessment of a patient with an abdominal injury, you observe protruded intestinal organs. His clothes are torn and soaked with blood and visceral tissues. What step of emergency management is incorrect?

A. Cut away any attached clothing.
B. Try to replace the intestines into the abdomen.
C. Place a pre-moistened dressing over the wound.
D. Place an occlusive dressing over a pre-moistened dressing.

111. Which of the following is not a form of male genitalia injury?

A. Avulsion
B. Laceration
C. Concussion
D. Contusion

112. Which of the following is not a form of injury to the female genitalia?

A. Avulsion
B. Laceration
C. Concussion
D. Contusion

113. A 10-year-old female sustained a straddle injury after a fall while playing in a park. On examination, a vulval laceration is observed. Which of the following assessment and management protocols is false for a female genitalia injury?

A. Apply direct pressure to stop any bleeding.
B. Having a female EMT attend to this patient is not important.
C. Consider applying a cold compress to reduce pain and swelling.
D. Save any avulsed or amputated tissue.

114. A patient was rushed to the emergency room with a fracture following a car crash. Which of the following mechanisms of injury is least important during the assessment?

A. Direct force
B. Indirect force
C. Twisting force
D. Rolling force

115. A 13-year-old male sustained a left elbow fracture following a fall on the arm while swinging in the school playground. Which of the following symptoms are not important to look out for?

A. Pain
B. Swelling
C. Deformity
D. Tenderness

116. A truck driver was involved in a motor vehicle crash. He was extracted from the car drowsy and is disoriented with midshaft (probably a spiral left tibial) fracture, head trauma, and bruises over his arms. Which of the following interventions is inappropriate?

A. Do not administer oxygen.
B. Give oxygen only when required.
C. Splint all injuries or fractures before transport.
D. Elevate the injured extremity.

117. On assessment of the other victim of the crash, you realize that he sustained a left midshaft femoral fracture. How should you not splint the patient's fracture before referral?

A. Immobilize the knee and hip joints.
B. Align with gentle traction before splinting.
C. Cover up the wound with a sterile dressing.
D. Move the patient before splinting the limb.

118. Patients with splinting may encounter certain complications. Which of the following is not a complication of splinting?

A. The neurovasculature and tissues may be compressed.
B. There may be reduced blood circulation to areas above the splint.
C. The splint may aggravate the injury.
D. The time it takes to splint the injury may delay transport of patients with life-threatening conditions.

119. Which of the following steps is incorrect in splinting a left midshaft femoral injury?

A. Manually apply stabilization.
B. Assess the pulse as well as motor and sensory innervation.
C. Immobilize only the site of injury.
D. Align with gentle traction if the distal femoral shaft is cyanotic.

120. Use of traction in splinting of orthopedic trauma injuries is contraindicated in all except which of the following?

A. Injuries at the ankle joints of the lower leg
B. Injuries at the hip joints or pelvis
C. A partially amputated or avulsed injury with bone separation
D. Midshaft injuries to long bones

Test 3: Answers and Explanations

1. (C) The patient will not require transportation once the seizure is aborted.
This statement is false concerning this patient's management. Although she has had previous seizures, the patient must be transported to the ER for medical investigation and diagnosis.

2. (C) Reduction of stridor is a good sign in children who have previously demonstrated signs of severe obstruction.
This statement is false. In children with croup, reduced stridor is an alarming sign because it points to worsening obstruction of the airway.

3. (C) Incidence has been reduced with the advent of a vaccine.
This statement is true. Epiglottitis is a bacterial infection usually caused by Hemophilus influenzae type B. With the advent of vaccines, its incidence has been reduced. Cases can be seen in adults who abuse cocaine. Symptoms include fever, hoarseness, drooling, and difficulty swallowing.

4. (A) The tongue and jaw are proportional.
This statement is false. The pediatric tongue is relatively large compared to the small mandible and can block the airway in an unconscious child.

5. (C) High-pitched snoring noise while inhaling
This is not a sign of mild airway obstruction. This describes stridor and is a sign of severe airway obstruction. A wheeze may also be a sign of severe airway obstruction.

6. (D) All of the above
Other factors that should be assessed include the effort of breathing, emotional state, response to the EMT, interaction with the environment, and tone/body position.

7. (D) All of the above
The PAT can help an EMT determine how critical a child's condition is before rushing right up to the child. You can begin a close-up assessment after performing PAT.

8. (C) Signs of trauma always appear early in the injury.
This statement is incorrect. A child may be injured and display no obvious early signs, so close monitoring is necessary.

9. (A) Lay the boy supine, commence supplemental oxygen, and give IV fluids if authorized while preparing him for transport.
The patient is most likely in septic shock and will benefit from effective oxygenation and fluid resuscitation. In septic shock there is widespread vasodilation leading to hypotension, so fluid resuscitation, especially in the first hour, is important. Early administration of antibiotics is also important, so the boy should be transported to the hospital promptly.

10. (D) Psychogenic shock
Psychogenic shock is the most likely cause of this girl's presentation. It is caused by an initial dilation of the blood vessels. This is followed by a drop in blood pressure and increased pulse rate. There is also a decrease in blood supply to the brain, causing a loss of consciousness.

11. (C) Anaphylaxis
Anaphylaxis presents with hypotension due to vasodilation, but this does not manifest as pallor. Flushing of the skin is seen in some cases.

12. (B) Continue CPR for two more minutes.
According to the algorithm for cardiac arrest in pediatric patients, if after administering one shock and delivering CPR for two minutes, you reassess and there is no shockable rhythm, you should continue with CPR for two more minutes, secure an IV/IO access if authorized, and give IV epinephrine.

13. (C) Pertussis
The history of paroxysmal cough, fever, thick mucoid expectoration, and deep breaths after each coughing episode (whoop) indicates a prehospital diagnosis of pertussis. Croup presents with a raspy cough and stridor. In epiglottitis, there is high fever and drooling. Pneumonia will present with cough, fever, anorexia, and rhonchi. Also, coughing spells in pneumonia are not prolonged.

14. (D) Administer humidified supplemental oxygen after taking universal precautions.
Giving supplemental humidified oxygen to relieve respiratory distress is appropriate in this case. Whooping cough is very contagious; therefore, you need to wear PPE, including a HEPA mask. Separating a child from the mother will not be helpful, as preschoolers have separation anxiety if removed from parents or caregivers. Oral acetaminophen can be given after respiratory distress is ameliorated. Clear the airway with a suction machine.

15. (C) Commence BVM ventilation.
An appropriate intervention would be to commence ventilation, since the child has no respiratory effort and a weak pulse. Giving ventilations early can reverse or prevent further deterioration of cardiopulmonary function. The patient has no respiratory effort, so giving oxygen through a nasal cannula will not be helpful. Although N-acetyl cysteine is the antidote for paracetamol poisoning, ventilation in this patient should be secured before commencement of the antidote.

16. (A) Help the patient into a comfortable position and suction.
Maintaining a position of comfort for the patient and suctioning is the most appropriate management to help clear the patient's airway. Supplemental oxygen can be given to maintain adequate oxygen saturation after suctioning. The oropharyngeal airway is not useful here and will make the patient gag. Oral mucolytics are not helpful, and the patient has to be stabilized before making transport arrangements.

17. (D) Chain of custody
Chain of custody is different documentation from a prehospital care report. It involves paperwork and documentation used to prove that forensic evidence has not been tampered with. Prehospital care report is used for continuity of care; to evaluate the quality of care; and for administrative, billing, and educational purposes.

18. (C) Have a family member sign in the patient's place.
If a patient refuses to sign the refusal form, have a police officer, bystander, or family member sign as a witness of the patient's refusal to sign.

19. (D) Patient education on counseling and psychotherapy services
This information is not required. It is not in the EMT's scope of practice to give information on counseling and psychotherapy services.

20. (D) Draw a single horizontal line through the error.
This is the most appropriate method of erasing the error. After drawing the line, add your initials on top and make the corrections. Covering the error with Wite-Out can give the impression that you are trying to cover up fraud or a mistake.

21. (D) It has a limited range.
This statement is correct. Portable receivers/transmitters are handheld devices with a very limited range. Mobile transmitters are two-way radios that are mounted on vehicles. They can transmit at values lower than that of base stations. Also, they cover a wider range than handheld transmitters.

22. (D) The patient's clinical state.
The patient's clinical state is information required for the physician to prescribe the drug to be used.

23. (C) Repeat the order back to the physician.
This is the most appropriate method of clarifying the dose of this drug. Writing the order on paper can waste time required to attend to this patient.

24. (C) Abandonment
You and your partner have demonstrated abandonment of this patient. You are expected to hand this patient over to the emergency nurse with your patient care report and any other report that can be useful in management. Under no circumstances are you to leave this patient without a proper handoff. The appropriate thing to do is to inform the dispatch officer of your unavailability to answer the call.

25. (D) Education of family members
An EMT cannot share a patient's health information with family members, friends, and even caregivers without permission/expressed consent from the patient.

26. (C) Incident command
The role of incident command is given to the response unit that arrives first at the incident. The team with incident command is responsible for assessing the incident and delegating tasks to other response units. This encourages collaboration and prevents waste of resources and time.

27. (C) Assess the safety of the location.
The incident commander is responsible for ensuring the safety of personnel and surviving victims. To do this, the immediate environment should first be assessed for potential hazards. In this case, the environment should be scanned for shooters and weapons. Usually, the environment ought to be cleared by the armed forces before emergency care is commenced.

28. (A) Ask patients who can stand to do so.
To begin START triage, locate the walking wounded. Do this by asking patients who can walk to stand up. After this, relocate them to a different area that is separate from the area set up for triage. These patients should be tagged with a green ribbon. After this, begin assessing the victims in the triage area according to respiration, circulation, and mental status. Move in a coordinated manner and keep track of the number of patients. Patients should be tagged with the appropriate color-coded ribbon.

29. (A) Red
Red tag (immediate) – Patients in this category require immediate treatment. Their cardiopulmonary function is compromised, and they are likely to die if they are not stabilized.

30. (C) Yellow
Yellow (delayed) – Patients in this category can have their treatment delayed for a few minutes until patients in the red category are stabilized.

31. (B) Black
Black (dead/cannot be helped) – Patients in this category have the least priority. These patients are either dead clinically or are in a state where resuscitation is of no benefit.

32. (D) All of the above
Downed electrical lines, explosions, and fire are all possible hazards at the scene of an accident. EMT personnel need to survey a scene and ensure their personal safety before rendering medical assistance.

33. (D) None of the above
All these items are essential to an EMT responding to a hazmat scene. The binoculars allow you to view and assess hazardous scenes from a distance. The emergency response guidebook provides a guide for first responders dealing with hazardous materials. Placards on buildings help in identifying hazardous substances.

34. (D) Scores are given based on verbal and motor responses and eye-opening.
This statement is true. GCS is used to evaluate the entire neurological function of a patient. Scores range from 3 to 15.

35. (B) Localizes pain – 4
This statement is incorrect. A patient who can localize pain is given a score of 5, while a score of 4 is given if the patient only withdraws from pain. A score of 3 is given if the patient flexes in response to pain.

36. (C) 10
The patient's total score on the Glasgow Coma Scale is 10. A score of 2 is assigned for eye opening to pain, while confused speech and ability to withdraw from pain are scored 4 each.

37. (A) Gag reflex is absent
Before administering oral glucose, first ensure that the patient's gag reflex is intact. This reduces the risk of aspiration.

38. (C) Beta-agonists
Beta-agonists are sympathomimetics. They increase the risk of hyperglycemia rather than hypoglycemia.

39. (D) None of the above.
Decreasing serum glucose, increasing glucose metabolism, and secretions from beta cells being stimulated by high glucose are all false concerning insulin. Some actions of insulin include increasing glucose transport into cells and stimulating glycogenolysis in the liver.

40. (D) Administering oral glucose
This intervention is inappropriate. Oral glucose should not be administered to this patient with a suspected hyperglycemic emergency. You should monitor and maintain his airway and other vital signs and transport him as quickly as possible.

41. (D) None of the above
The length of the coma, onset of the coma, and/or a history of drug abuse are not necessary information in assessing this patient. Important information includes a history of recent head trauma, current medical history, and history of use of medical alert tags.

42. (D) All of the above
Head trauma, stroke, and sepsis all may be responsible for this presentation. Other causes of altered mental status include acidosis, alcohol abuse, medication overdose, uremia, and psychosis.

43. (D) None of the above
All the listed factors can alter a patient's behavior. Other factors include low blood sugar, lack of oxygen, head trauma, and mind-altering substances.

44. (C) A 36-year-old female who is married and has flexible work hours
This person has the lowest risk of suicide. Risk factors of suicidal/self-destructive behaviors include previous history of self-harm; an unusual collection of articles that can cause death, including pills, guns, and other weapons; and having little social support and/or being single, widowed, or divorced. Persons recently diagnosed with serious illness or who have recently lost a loved one are also at risk of suicide.

45. (D) All of the above
Knowing whether the patient has suicidal tendencies, whether any interventions have been given, and how the patient feels are all factors that will determine if there is a need to call for external help and, if so, who needs to be called. Other questions to be considered include if the patient is a threat to himself or others.

46. (B) The patient may be left alone for no more than 10 minutes.
This statement is false. As much as possible, a patient who is at risk of self-harm should not be left alone.

47. (D) Amnesic psychogenic dissociative disorder
This is the most likely diagnosis. In this condition, a person is unable to remember personal information following severe psychological stress; however, the person is usually calm and can recall other memories.

48. (D) None of the above
It is always important to note that an intoxicated patient may exhibit unexpected violent or disruptive behavior, have abnormal responses to physical problems, or give a faulty history. Responders should be alert and able to tie signs/symptoms to the history taken.

49. (B) Cogentin
Cogentin (benztropine mesylate) is used to treat dystonia in patients. Drugs that may precipitate this condition include haloperidol, Thorazine, and Compazine.

50. (A) On no occasion should force be applied.
This statement is false. A "reasonable amount" depends on what force is necessary to keep a patient from injuring themself or others. It is determined by the patient's sex, size, and strength; type of abnormal behavior; mental state; and method of restraint.

51. (D) Avoiding reasonable force when indicated
This will not help protect an EMT against false accusations. In actuality, not using reasonable force when it is called for may be detrimental to the patient/responder. Having same-sex attendants/third-party witnesses may come in handy, especially if an EMT is accused of sexual misconduct.

52. (A) Packing the vaginal canal with a dressing
No attempt should be made to pack the vaginal canal, as this may trigger further bleeding. A large absorbable pad may be placed at the vaginal opening while other supportive measures are carried out.

53. (B) Ectopic pregnancy
There should be a high suspicion of ectopic pregnancy in patients with missed periods who experience vaginal bleeding and abdominal pain. Some forms of miscarriage may also present in this way.

54. (B) Having a trusted friend or family member present
As much as possible, a patient should be interviewed in the absence of family members. Attention should be given to a patient's privacy and confidentiality when gathering a history.

55. (C) Menopause
A diagnosis of menopause is likely with the presenting symptoms in a patient who is older than 50. If she is less than 40, it is referred to as premature (early) menopause. A diagnosis of premature ovarian failure is made for females who have menopausal symptoms and are younger than 35.

56. (B) Dysmenorrhea
Dysmenorrhea is the most likely diagnosis. It involves severe pain and cramping during menstruation that interferes with normal daily functions. It is usually present in females younger than 20 due to increased prostaglandin secretion during ovulatory cycles. Secondary causes include endometriosis, adenomyosis, cervical stenosis, and pelvic adhesions.

57. (B) Pelvic inflammatory disease
This is the most likely diagnosis. Indicators of pelvic inflammatory disease in this patient include the presenting symptoms (abdominal pain, fever, vaginal discharge, nausea, and vomiting) and a history of unprotected sexual intercourse with multiple sexual partners.

58. (C) Hepatitis A
Hepatitis A is not a sexually transmitted disease. It is transmitted primarily via the feco-oral route. Symptoms include fatigue, abdominal pain, nausea, and low-grade fever.

59. (B) Hyperventilation syndrome
The woman most likely has hyperventilation syndrome, which is ventilation above the body's metabolic requirements. Deep and rapid breathing leads to a reduction in SaO_2, which causes paresthesia, tetany dizziness, headaches, and visual disturbances. Acute respiratory distress syndrome, acute asthmatic attacks, and acute coronary syndrome are not associated with deep rapid breathing and paresthesia.

60. (D) Blood-clotting disorders
Blood-clotting disorders are nonmodifiable risk factors for pulmonary embolism. Clotting disorders, such as factor V LEIDEN, make the blood prone to abnormal clotting. Combined oral contraceptives, obesity, and smoking are all modifiable risk factors for pulmonary embolism because lifestyle modifications can improve these risks.

61. (A) Acute pulmonary embolism
Acute pulmonary embolism is the most likely prehospital diagnosis, given the history of dyspnea, cough, shortness of breath, and recent femoral neck repair. Reduced oxygen concentration also indicates hypoxia from pulmonary embolism. In pneumonia, affected patients have fever, cough, and sputum. Angina pectoris and myocardial infarction present with acute chest pain.

62. (A) Secure the child's airway and establish adequate ventilation.
Smoke inhalation and burns can cause swelling in the airway and laryngeal edema, which affect ventilation. Carbon monoxide poisoning can also occur in this condition, leading to unconsciousness and even death. Hence, securing the airway and commencing effective ventilation is of utmost priority. Providing emergency transport is important; however, this should not deter prompt airway management. Taking a detailed history will slow the patient's management and should be done only once the patient is stabilized. This also applies to reassuring the child's parents.

63. (B) Pulmonary edema
Pulmonary edema is the most likely prehospital diagnosis for this patient, as it can present with sudden onset of shortness of breath. Obesity, hypertension, and COPD are risk factors present in this patient. Bilateral pedal edema, reduced oxygen saturation, crackles, and reduced air bilaterally all point to alveolar congestion. In pulmonary embolism, edema is usually unilateral with a history of chest pain and may often look cyanosed. Acute respiratory distress syndrome and bronchiolitis are unlikely.

64. (D) Insert a nasogastric suction tube.
Inserting a nasogastric suction tube helps aspirate air contents and decompress the stomach. This will improve ventilation. Gastric distension splints the diaphragm and reduces the efficiency of ventilation. Use of a nasopharyngeal airway is indicated in semi-conscious patients to prevent the tongue from falling back and blocking the airway. Reposition the head if the chest is not rising and falling with ventilations. Create a tighter seal on the mask if the air is escaping from the face mask.

65. (D) All of the above
Sinusitis, recent nasal surgery, esophageal varices, and maxillofacial trauma are all contraindications to insertion of a NG tube. The tube may introduce infections that may be fatal or rupture existing esophageal varices.

66. (B) Bronchodilators
Bronchodilators are drugs that dilate the bronchial tubes to decrease resistance in the respiratory airway and airflow to the lungs. They include anticholinergic bronchodilators; theophylline; and beta-agonists, such as albuterol, formoterol, and salbutamol. Mucolytics thin out mucus and make it easy to expel. Corticosteroids and mast stabilizers are used in asthma management. However, they do not primarily dilate the airway.

67. (A) Nasopharyngeal airway
The nasopharyngeal airway is less likely to stimulate gag reflex and vomiting in a patient with an intact reflex. This makes it suitable for use in responsive patients who need assistance in keeping the tongue from obstructing the airway. The oropharyngeal airway is used to prevent the tongue from blocking the airway in patients who are unconscious and have no gag reflex. Endotracheal and nasogastric tubes are not used for this purpose.

68. (A) Measure from the corner of the patient's lips to the ramus of the mandible.
To select a proper-sized oropharyngeal airway, measure from the corner of the patient's lips to the ramus of the mandible or the earlobe. This tells you the appropriate size of the airway to b use.

69. (B) Jaw thrust
A jaw thrust is used to open up the airway when a spinal injury is suspected or when the patient has an unknown mechanism of injury. This is to prevent worsening any cervical spine or cranial nerve injuries. A head-tilt/chin-lift is used when there are no suspected cervical spine injuries. The log-rolling technique is used when an unconscious patient produces so much emesis that it cannot be adequately suctioned. A chin sweep lift is not used in opening the airway for artificial ventilation.

70. (A) The nose
Infant breathing mainly depends on the nose. Infants struggle to breathe through the mouth if the nose is congested or obstructed. Children are considered obligate nose breathers, so suctioning a secretion-filled nasopharynx can improve breathing problems in an infant.

71. (A) Hypoxic drive
In hypoxic drive, the body uses oxygen chemoreceptors to regulate the respiratory cycle. The primary stimulus for breathing is the amount of CO_2, but in hypoxic drive, decreased oxygen levels provide a stimulus for breathing. This occurs in a small percentage of COPD patients.

72. (D) All of the above
The tongue, foreign body, trauma, infections, burns, and allergic reactions are all causes of airway compromise.

73. (A) Remove the device from the patient, turn off the valve, and remove all pressure from the regulator.
The correct operating procedure when oxygen use is complete is to remove the device from the patient, turn off the valve, and remove all pressure from the regulator.

74. (A) Tension pneumothorax
Tension pneumothorax should be suspected if, after blunt chest injury, there is sudden dyspnea, tracheal deviation, absent or reduced breath sounds, and hyperresonant percussion notes. Myocardial infarction, flail chest syndrome, and acute chest syndrome do not cause tracheal deviation.

75. (A) Pulmonary artery
Occlusion of the pulmonary artery leads to an interruption of the blood supply to the lungs. The pulmonary veins and the inferior and superior vena cava do not supply blood directly to the lungs; hence, this will not cause occlusion of the blood supply to the lungs.

76. (A) Provide supplemental oxygen.
The scenario is indicative of diabetic ketoacidosis. Supplemental oxygen will help improve oxygen saturation, as the patient is hypoxic. Random blood glucose can be determined after ventilatory support is given. Breathing into a paper bag will cause CO_2 retention. Chest compressions are not indicated.

77. (D) Give supplemental oxygen with a non-rebreather mask.
The patient's symptoms are suggestive of pneumonia. The non-rebreather mask will supply high-flow oxygen and improve the patient's oxygen saturation. A Venturi mask, nasal cannula, and blow-by technique will not provide the high oxygen concentrations necessary for improving the patient's hypoxia.

78. (A) Assist the patient into an upright position with his feet dangling for comfort.
This case scenario is suggestive of congestive cardiac failure. An upright position with the feet dangling will help relieve the patient's pulmonary congestion and improve symptoms of orthopnea. Supplemental oxygen should be administered. The lateral recovery position, rescue inhaler, and humidified oxygen are not helpful in this patient.

79. (D) All of the above
Continuous positive airway pressure is indicated in cardiogenic pulmonary edema, hypoxic respiratory failure, and obstructive sleep apnea. It delivers constant positive airway pressure at a level greater than atmospheric pressure and aids in keeping the alveoli open, thereby improving oxygen saturation levels.

80. (A) Stridor is a high-pitched harsh sound heard on inspiration.
This statement is true regarding abnormal breath sounds. Stridor is a sign of upper airway obstruction. It is heard only on inspiration.

81. (A) A permanent artificial opening in the trachea
A tracheostomy is a permanent artificial opening made in the trachea to open the airway and aid breathing. An opening in the larynx is called a laryngectomy.

82. (C) HbAC
HbAC patients are phenotypically normal. Clinical manifestations occur only when the hemoglobin C is in combination with HbS.

83. (D) Performing chest compressions and ventilations at a ratio of 30:2
Simultaneous chest compressions and ventilation are administered as 30 chest compressions followed by two ventilations.

84. (B) Sepsis
The patient's presentation is most likely sepsis from the improperly treated right knee bruise. The microbes have migrated into the man's bloodstream, causing the widespread systemic manifestations he is presenting with.

85. (A) Take over applying pressure, elevate the woman's hands, wrap a pressure dressing around the wound, and transport her to a hospital.
Use sterile gauze over the wounds and apply pressure with gloved hands. Elevating the limb and pressure dressings also augment hemorrhage control. It is essential to check for pulses distal and proximal to the pressure dressing to ensure it is not too tight. If these are not effective, pressure points can then be occluded in addition to the above and not in isolation.

86. (B) Aortic aneurysm
Aortic aneurysms are dilatations in any part of the aorta. Thoracic aneurysms sometimes compress surrounding structures, like the esophagus and trachea, affecting swallowing and breathing.

87. (C) Administer IV or IO epinephrine immediately and give supplemental oxygen.
Epinephrine is the most effective drug for anaphylaxis. The patient most likely has a penicillin allergy, even if he is not aware of this. Steroids and antihistamines can be given later, but they are not immediate in action and are therefore unsuitable for emergencies.

88. (A) Place him in a comfortable position, administer supplemental oxygen, and carry out an ECG.
Calming the patient's anxiety is important. Then supplemental oxygen should be given to increase saturation. An ECG should then be carried out to ascertain if it is an MI. Both MI and angina patients should be treated alike.

89. (A) Lay the woman supine, commence CPR, and transport her to the hospital immediately.
This is the most appropriate intervention. The woman most likely is in cardiogenic shock with pulmonary edema.

90. (C) Chest pain with a blood pressure of 132/70 mmHg with a doctor's prescription of nitroglycerin
Nitroglycerin is most likely indicated in the patient in Option C. This is because nitroglycerin should not be given when a person's systolic blood pressure is less than 100 mmHg.

91. (D) Administer a shock while your partner is administering rescue breaths.
This is not one of the steps of using an AED. You should always clear the patient before administering shocks.

92. (D) Neurogenic shock
The patient most likely has a cervical spine injury, which can cause neurogenic shock. This explains the hypotension and bradycardia. If the damage is below the C5 vertebrae, it can cause diaphragmatic breathing.

93. (C) Aortic aneurysm
A stabbing, piercing, or knife-like pain in the chest, usually behind the sternum, is indicative of an aortic aneurysm or dissection.

94. (A) Administer supplemental oxygen and the man's prescribed nitroglycerin, perform an ECG, and transport him to a hospital.
The man's prescribed nitroglycerin points to the fact that he has a history of chest pain. Both MI and angina should be managed similarly in the field. You should administer supplemental oxygen and the man's prescribed nitroglycerin, perform an ECG, and transport him to a hospital quickly.

95. (A) Lay the man in the Trendelenburg position, commence supplemental oxygen, and transport him to a hospital.
This is the most appropriate intervention. The man has most likely developed anemia, possibly from his new vegetarian diet.

96. (B) Administer another shock to a maximum of three shocks if VF persists.
A maximum of three shocks is advised in order to identify and treat shockable rhythms as quickly as possible.

97. (B) Stop the vehicle if heart rhythm analysis is necessary and deliver a shock if needed.
When using an AED, you should stop the vehicle to analyze the heart rhythm and shock as indicated.

98. (A) Hypertensive urgency
Hypertensive urgency is severely elevated blood pressure without any evidence of target organ damage, with some literature using the cut-off of 180/110 mmHg. It may present with headaches, shortness of breath, anxiety, etc.

99. (D) Dehydration
Dehydration can arise from frequent loose stools.

100. (C) Anaphylaxis
Anaphylaxis is the most likely cause. Urticaria describes the skin condition caused by anaphylaxis. This patient has both urticaria and angioedema, which are symptoms of anaphylaxis.

101. (C) Epinephrine
Epinephrine is most effective in treating anaphylaxis. Early administration is essential.

102. (D) Remove the object from the opposite direction and pack both sides of the wound.
This statement is false. Impaled objects compromising airflow or airway patency should always be removed in the direction of entry to avoid further injury to the tissues and consequent worsening of respiratory activity. Both sides of the cheeks should be packed after removal.

103. (D) Decreased heart rate with warm and moist skin
This mechanism of injury does not explain what may happen to a patient with an open chest injury after an encounter with armed robbers. Apart from a possible lung collapse following pneumothorax and hemothorax, the patient will have labored breathing with pale, cool, dry skin, as well as an increased heart rate.

104. (A) Costochondritis
Costochondritis is an inflammation of the rib cartilage and is unlikely after a closed chest injury. All other answer options are effects of traumatic chest injury with air trapped within the thoracic and pleural spaces following rib fractures. Patients usually present with respiratory distress and will need advanced respiratory support.

105. (D) Decreased or absent breath sounds on the affected side
This statement is correct regarding a pneumothorax. Breath sounds are reduced or absent on the affected side. There is tracheal deviation to the unaffected side. Other signs are equal chest rise and jugular venous distension, which is a late sign.

106. (B) Ensure airway patency with a chin tilt irrespective of suspected cervical injury.
To maintain airway patency, a jaw-thrust maneuver (not a chin tilt) should be done in suspected cases of coexisting cervical spinal injury. With chest injuries, airway, breathing, and circulation may be compromised depending on severity.

107. (B) Removing any impaled object from the patient
Removal of objects impaled in the chest is contraindicated because it increases the risk of bleeding and tamponade. The right step is to stabilize the object.

108. (D) Tracheal deviation
Tracheal deviation is not a chest injury in itself but is a sign of chest injuries, like tension pneumothorax. Also, it is not a life-threatening condition, unlike injuries like flail segment with consequent lung collapse.

109. (A) Transport the patient from the scene immediately, irrespective of safety.
This step is incorrect because the scene can give a clue to the mechanism of injury, such as if it is a vehicle collision, blunt injury, or penetrating stab injury. It is also necessary to allow ample time to access other possible victims.

110. (B) Try to replace the intestines into the abdomen.
This step of emergency management is incorrect. After an abdominal injury, any protruded or eviscerated organ should not be touched or pushed back into the abdomen, as this increases the risk of infections, peritonitis, and sepsis.

111. (C) Concussion
A concussion is not a form of male genitalia injury. It is a brain injury from a blow or a shaking of the head, with or without loss of consciousness. There is cognitive impairment.

112. (C) Concussion
This is not a form of female genitalia injury. A concussion is a brain injury from a blow or a shaking of the head, with or without loss of consciousness. There is cognitive impairment

113. (B) Having a female EMT attend to this patient is not important.
This statement is false. It is very important to have a female EMT attend to this patient to provide a sense of privacy, empathy, and care.

114. (D) Rolling force
A rolling force will likely not cause an orthopedic injury and is not a mechanism of injury that is vital during assessment. Most orthopedic traumatic injuries occur via direct force of the moving object on the body and indirect transferable impact or a sudden external force, causing an involuntary twisting of the body with resultant trauma to tissue and fracture to impacted bony surface.

115. (D) Tenderness
Tenderness is not a symptom that is important to look out for. Rather, it is a sign elicited on examination of patients. It is also a sign of orthopedic trauma injury. Along with pain and swelling, the range of motion at the elbow joint is limited. An ulnar fracture is common.

116. (A) Do not administer oxygen.
This intervention is inappropriate. Depending on the severity, the patient's respiratory function may be compromised. Assessment of airway patency and flow is crucial. If indicated, oxygen therapy is very important in assisting the patient's ventilation.

117. (D) Move the patient before splinting the limb.
This intervention is inappropriate. You should first immobilize the joints above and below the injury. Align with gentle traction, especially if there is a deformity, then dress the wound before splinting. After this, you may move the patient. Splinting limits further soft tissue injury by reducing the mobility of the affected limb.

118. (B) There may be reduced blood circulation to areas above the splint.
This is not a complication of splinting. Due to compression of blood vessels at the splint, there may be reduced blood flow to regions below the splint and tissue hypoxia. This cannot happen above the splint since the blood supply above is not compromised. In cases of coexisting multiple rib fractures and limb fractures, the ribs can cause closed chest injuries with breathing difficulties.

119. (C) Immobilize only the site of injury.
This statement is incorrect. The joints above and below the injury should always be immobilized—not only the site of injury. Also, assess the pulse and innervations before and after splinting. Apply gentle traction to avoid compressing blood supply distal to the point of splinting.

120. (D) Midshaft injuries to long bones
A traction splint is not contraindicated in midshaft injuries to long bones. Its use is not beneficial in joint fractures. Partially amputated or avulsed injuries are at risk of separation if such a splint is used. When splinting, gentle traction should be applied to avoid neurovascular vessel compression, which can decrease sensation, circulation, and oxygenation to tissues below the splint.

Test 4: Questions

1. According to START triage, which of the following patients should be attended to first?
   A. A teenage female with a closed fracture of the right arm, RR 22 cpm, capillary refill less than two seconds, can obey commands, crying and distressed
   B. An adult male with an open fracture to the thigh, cool and clammy skin, radial pulse absent, RR 30 cpm
   C. An elderly male with no respiratory effort after a modified jaw thrust
   D. An adult female with amputation of the left foot, distressed, obeys commands, RR 25 cpm, capillary refill more than two seconds

2. Which of the following is not a feature of red-tag patients according to START triage?
   A. RR less than 30 cpm
   B. Capillary refill less than two seconds
   C. Altered mental status
   D. Absent radial pulse

3. Concerning START triage, which of the following is false?
   A. Circulation is assessed first.
   B. Patients with a black tag are the least prioritized.
   C. Patients with a green tag are moved out of the triage area.
   D. Patients with a red tag have an impalpable radial pulse.

4. When triaging, it is best to do which of the following?
   A. Start from the unconscious patients.
   B. Start from the bleeding patients.
   C. Start from where you are.
   D. Start with children.

5. You have been dispatched to a location exposed to hazardous materials. Part of your initial job is to size up the location and confirm the presence of hazardous materials. Which of the following resources is not useful in confirming hazardous materials?
   A. DOT placards
   B. UN numbers
   C. MSDS
   D. OSHA

6. Which of the following is correct about the hot zone in a hazmat scene?
   A. It is also known as the decontamination zone.
   B. Access with Level A PPE is required.
   C. The risk of secondary contamination is very high.
   D. PPE requires air-purifying respirators.

7. Which of the following is correct about the warm zone?
   A. The risk of primary contamination is high.
   B. Access with Level C PPE is required.
   C. The PPE must contain air-purifying respirators.
   D. It is not accessible to health personnel.

8. Which of the following is correct about the cold zone?
   A. It is also called the decontamination zone.
   B. There is a risk of secondary contamination.
   C. Standard precautions are sufficient in protecting personnel.
   D. Level B PPE is required.

9. Concerning secondary contamination, which of the following is false?
   A. Gases are common sources of secondary contamination.
   B. It can spread via contaminated clothes.
   C. Exposed patients must pass through the warm zone before they receive emergency care.
   D. Contamination is indirect.

10. Which of the following is a rare mode of decontamination?
   A. Neutralization
   B. Dilution
   C. Disposal
   D. Absorption

11. You are responding to a mass casualty incident caused by exposure to a nerve agent. You expect victims to demonstrate all except which of the following symptoms?
   A. Rhinorrhea
   B. Diarrhea
   C. Miosis
   D. Urinary retention

12. You arrive at a recreational park where a chemical agent has been released. You notice a group of people coughing and covering their noses with their clothes. You also notice two bleeding victims on the ground. Which of the following interventions is most appropriate?

A. Park your vehicle at a safe distance.
B. Tell the coughing victims to leave the scene.
C. Commence external compression on the bleeding victims.
D. Tell the coughing victims to take off their clothes.

13. A group of patients who have been exposed to mustard gas will experience all except which of the following symptoms?

A. Cough
B. Lacrimation
C. Skin blisters
D. Diarrhea

14. Your response team is approaching a mass casualty incident where hydrogen sulfide was released. Which of the following mechanisms is responsible for the symptoms in the victims?

A. Irritation of the respiratory mucosa
B. Skin blisters
C. Inhibition of acetylcholinesterase
D. Cellular anoxia

15. Which of the following is correct about Level B protection?

A. It gives a high level of eye protection.
B. It gives a high level of skin protection.
C. It gives a high level of respiratory protection.
D. It is made of chemical-resistant material.

16. What level of protection is provided by a firefighter's uniform?

A. A
B. B
C. C
D. D

17. Your team has arrived at a mass casualty scene where victims have been exposed to anthrax. Which of the following is false about anthrax?

A. It is a biological agent.
B. It can spread via contact, inhalation, and ingestion.
C. It is caused by spores from aerobic bacteria.
D. The incubation period of the inhaled spores is longer than that from contact contamination.

18. Which of the following is the most common route of dissemination of biological weapons?

A. Food
B. Contact
C. Aerosol
D. Water

19. Which of the following toxins is not considered a threat by the CDC?

A. Botulinum toxin
B. Tetanus toxin
C. Epsilon toxin
D. Ricin toxin

20. Your team is responding to a group of people exposed to botulinum toxin in an abortion clinic. You expect manifestations of all except which of the following symptoms?

A. Excessive salivation
B. Slurred speech
C. Drooping eyelids
D. Double vision

21. A 2-year-old child who is small for her age was brought to the children's emergency unit with symptoms of chills and rigors. A provisional diagnosis of hypothermia was made. Which of the following is not a possible predisposing factor for hypothermia in this child?

A. Cold environment
B. Immersion
C. Large surface area compared to the overall size
D. Small surface area compared to the overall size

22. Unlike adults, there are physiological changes in children that reduce their potential of being able to generate or conserve heat within the body. Which of the following physiological features does not support this tendency?

A. Small body mass
B. Less body fat
C. Well-developed ability to shiver during cold
D. Inability to put on clothes without assistance

23. A 66-year-old known diabetic with a 2-year history of recurrent cough was brought to the emergency room because of burns from a domestic accident. On examination, the woman is in shock. Which of the following medical conditions is least likely to worsen her risk for shock?

A. Hypoperfusion
B. Burns
C. Chronic cough
D. Diabetes

24. You were called by a colleague to see a 37-year-old male with hypothermia. In eliciting a history, what is the least likely symptom you should look out for?

A. Reduced tactile sensation
B. Dizziness
C. Stiff or rigid posture
D. Low blood pressure

25. After obtaining a history of the above patient, what is the least likely sign you expect to see in this patient on examination?

A. Joint pain
B. Sluggish pupillary movement
C. Cyanotic skin
D. Poor coordination

26. Assuming you were the first EMT to attend to the above patient, what is the least likely step you should take?

A. If the patient is unresponsive, massage his extremities.
B. Replace any wet clothing with dry clothes.
C. Administer humidified oxygen.
D. Before starting CPR, assess the pulse for about a minute.

27. For patients who are alert and responsive, which of the following steps in emergency management is incorrect?

A. Replace clothing with warm blankets.
B. Increase the heat around the patient.
C. Apply heat packs to the axillary, cervical, and inguinal regions.
D. Restrict oral intake even if the patient can tolerate it.

28. A 34-year-old female had a localized cold injury on her nose and right ear 15 minutes before presentation at the emergency room. You are unlikely to see which of the following on examination?

A. Loss of sensation on the right ear and nose
B. Soft skin over the injured region
C. Blisters
D. Blanching of skin

29. Assuming the above patient presented four hours later from the onset of a deep cold injury, all except which of the following signs may be present?

A. Frozen or fresh feeling on palpation
B. Tingling sensation
C. Swelling
D. Blisters

30. Which of the following emergency management protocols is incorrect pertaining to the patient above?

A. You should replace all wet or cold clothing with warm and dry clothes.
B. You should administer oxygen.
C. You should cover or splint the injured extremity if it is early or superficial.
D. You should massage or rub the injury.

31. All except which of the following factors can predispose infants or newborns to heat injury?

A. Low relative humidity in children
B. Poor thermoregulatory activity
C. Inability to remove clothing
D. Inability to move away from hot environments

32. Patients with extensive heat injury will likely present with all except which of the following symptoms?

A. Bradycardia
B. Exhaustion
C. Syncope
D. Unresponsiveness

33. You and your partner responded to a call for a patient with heatstroke. On arrival, you see that the patient is unconscious and covered in vomit. Which of the following positions is most appropriate in this patient?

A. Supine position
B. Left lateral position
C. Supine position with legs elevated
D. Position plays no role in the management

34. Though the incidence of cat bites is lower compared to dogs, what are the infection rates for cat bites?

A. 15% to 20%
B. 20% to 30%
C. 30% to 40%
D. 40% to 50%

35. Which of the following mammals have the most infectious bites?

A. Dog
B. Cat
C. Human
D. Bedbug

36. Concerning cat bites, which of the following is untrue?

A. They are usually on the arms and hands.
B. They usually leave behind a deep puncture wound.
C. They are mostly more infectious than dog bites.
D. Cat-scratch disease is life threatening.

37. A 12-year-old female has just been bitten on the back by a spider. The region is swollen with two red puncture marks. After some time, the patient experiences abdominal cramps. Which of the following is not a symptom of a bite from the black widow spider?

A. Tissue necrosis
B. Excessive sweating
C. Vertigo
D. Headache and breathing difficulties

38. All except which of the following are correct about snakebites?

A. Though painful, bites by coral snakes may be difficult to see.
B. In some bites, pit vipers may fail to envenomate their prey.
C. Venomous bites by pit vipers cause swelling after an hour.
D. Paralysis can occur from the sixth to fourteenth day.

39. A 4-year-old female was brought to the emergency room following a snakebite. Which of these responses is inappropriate?

A. Wash the area of the bite carefully.
B. Ensure cold is not applied to the snakebite.
C. Monitor the patient closely for symptoms and signs.
D. If the stinger is still present, you should scrape it out with forceps.

40. According to the AHA, which of the following is not part of the chain of survival for successful resuscitation?

A. Early CPR
B. Early defibrillation
C. Integrated post-cardiac arrest care
D. Deferred access

41. A 54-year-old hypertensive female experiences excruciating tearing pain in her chest and back, which started suddenly while she was making dinner. Her blood pressure is 98/70 mmHg with a pulse rate of 122 bpm and shortness of breath. What is your next line of action?

A. Lay the woman in a supine position, administer oxygen by intranasal cannula, perform an ECG, and quickly transport the patient to the hospital.
B. Sit the patient on a chair, administer supplemental oxygen, and commence IV fluids.
C. Commence rescue breaths and transport the patient to the hospital as quickly as possible.
D. Administer nitroglycerin and supplemental oxygen, then move the patient to the vehicle for transportation,

42. A 55-year-old female has been experiencing pain from urination, urge incontinence for about two weeks, fever, and nausea. She suddenly starts talking irrationally. She is pale with cold extremities. Her blood pressure is 86/65 mmHg, and she has a heart rate of 124 bpm. She has a respiratory rate of 28 cpm. What is the appropriate intervention?

A. Place the patient in a supine position and commence supplemental oxygen.
B. Sit the patient in a chair and commence supplemental oxygen.
C. Lay the patient in the Trendelenburg position and administer oxygen.
D. Strap the patient to the stretcher and administer oxygen.

43. You are carrying out an initial assessment on a patient with stabbing chest pain when you notice his blood pressure is 160/60 mmHg with a radial pulse of 26 bpm but no palpable pedal pulses. Which of the following is most likely the cause of this presentation?

A. Angina pectoris
B. Dehydration
C. Aortic aneurysm
D. Sepsis

44. Which of the following conditions is least likely to cause chest pain?

A. Stable angina
B. Anaphylaxis
C. Aortic aneurysm
D. Cardiogenic shock

45. You are about to administer CPR to a young male in cardiac arrest. Which of the following is not important for high-quality CPR?

A. Begin CPR with ventilation, not compressions.
B. For two-person CPR, deliver 2 breaths to 15 compressions.
C. As soon as AED pads are applied, stop everyone and activate the AED.
D. Depth of chest compressions should be at least two inches.

46. You are attending to a 49-year-old male who suddenly started gasping for air with dizziness and sweating. You find him sitting on the floor against a wall, feverish, with a pulse rate of 103 bpm, blood pressure of 98/70 mmHg, and respiratory rate of 34 cpm. He has been having painful urination for the past three weeks and is yet to see a doctor. What is the most appropriate intervention?

A. Administer analgesics for the man's pain.
B. Lay the man in a supine position, assess his saturation, and give supplemental oxygen if needed.
C. Commence the man on broad-spectrum antibiotics,
D. Hydrate the man with oral fluids and commence supplemental oxygen.

47. A 77-year-old female experiences anxiety, weakness, and confusion. She complains of shortness of breath that is worse when she lies down. Her blood pressure is 97/65 mmHg, and her skin is cool. Her respiratory rate is 30 cpm, with an oxygen saturation of 90% and crepitations heard on auscultation. What is the most likely cause of the woman's difficulty breathing?

A. Sepsis
B. Anaphylaxis
C. Pulmonary edema in cardiogenic shock
D. Congestive cardiac failure

48. You are administering nitroglycerin to a 43-year-old male with chest pain. Which of the following is a common side effect you should look out for?

A. Hypotension
B. Hypoxia
C. Toxic epidermal necrolysis
D. Glaucoma

49. Which of the following is not included in medications used by EMTs in cardiovascular emergencies?

A. Epinephrine
B. Oxygen
C. Nitroglycerine
D. Furosemide

50. Your unit is called to an accident scene where a truck ran into a sedan at an intersection. You arrive to find the sole occupant of the sedan has been pulled out of the car and is lying unconscious in what appears to be a little less than three pints of her blood. What stage of hypovolemia is the woman in?

A. Stage 1
B. Stage 2
C. Stage 3
D. Stage 4

51. You are assessing a 42-year-old female in shock. Which one of these is not a manifestation of reduction in cerebral blood flow?

A. Agitation
B. Confusion
C. Vomiting
D. Unresponsiveness

52. You are called to a university campus where a student suddenly became unconscious during a class. You find him lying supine on the floor. His eyes are open, but he is confused. The patient's friend says he has been vomiting since the previous day after they got dinner from a food truck. He has vomited up to 10 times this morning alone. His blood pressure is 96/59 mmHg with a weak pulse of 118 bpm. His extremities are cold, and he is dyspneic. What is the most likely cause of this presentation?

A. Sepsis
B. Dehydration
C. DIC
D. Aortic dissection

53. A 40-year-old female presents with rashes on her hands and forearm, which she says began while she was cleaning her bathroom with a new type of latex gloves she just bought. She also complains of difficulty breathing, hoarseness, and her throat closing up. What is the most likely cause of this presentation?

A. Anaphylaxis
B. Sepsis
C. Asthma
D. Steven Johnson's syndrome

54. You are called to a building site on a hot day where a new construction worker has passed out. When you get there, he is lying on the floor with dry skin and lips, heart rate of 160 bpm, and blood pressure of 90/62 mmHg. His rectal temperature is 41° C. Which of the following will the patient most benefit from?

A. Supplemental oxygen
B. Cold-water immersion
C. Oral hydration
D. Smelling salts

55. You are called to an apartment complex where a 51-year-old hypertensive, diabetic and overweight male suddenly developed chest pain with shortness of breath and diaphoresis. Which of the following conditions can present like this?

A. Myocardial infarction
B. Septic shock
C. Constipation
D. Dehydration

56. You are administering CPR to a 33-year-old female in cardiac arrest. How deep should your chest compressions be?

A. Two inches
B. Half of the AP diameter of the chest
C. Two centimeters
D. Two-thirds of the AP diameter of the chest

57. While administering shocks to a patient with ventricular fibrillation, what is the maximum number of shocks that can be administered for a shockable rhythm before CPR can be recommenced?

A. Two
B. One
C. Three
D. Four

58. While carrying out an initial assessment on a patient suspected to be in cardiac arrest, how long should it take to check for breathing and pulse?

A. 10 minutes
B. 10 seconds
C. 5 minutes
D. 1 minute

59. Your unit is called to attend to a 54-year-old hypertensive male who developed chest pain with difficulty in breathing, weakness, and diaphoresis. His respiratory rate is 40 cpm with SPO2 of 86% and crackles on auscultation. His blood pressure is 82/56mm Hg, and his pulse rate is 128 bpm. What is your next course of action?

A. Lay the man in a supine position and administer supplemental oxygen.
B. Carry out an ECG and apply AED pads.
C. Place the man in the cardiac position and administer supplemental oxygen.
D. Place the man in the Trendelenburg position, keep him warm, and administer oxygen.

60. What kind of shock is most commonly seen with cervical spine injury?

A. Hypovolemic
B. Psychogenic
C. Neurogenic
D. Septic

61. You are commencing CPR for a 12-year-old female in cardiac arrest. Which of the following is not a component of high-quality CPR?

A. After each chest compression, allow the chest to recoil completely.
B. Perform a rhythm check every 10 minutes, lasting no more than 10 seconds.
C. A single rescuer can perform CPR with a compression to ventilation ratio of 30:2 and for two rescuers, a ratio of 15:2.
D. A chest compression rate of 100:120 in a minute is reasonable.

62. You are called to the scene of an accident where a 15-year-old male who was seated in the passenger seat of a car that was involved in a head-on collision with an SUV was thrown through the windshield onto the road. You find the patient lying face-up on the road, unconscious, with grunting respiration and a heart rate of 120 bpm. You must provide rescue breathing. Which of the following is most appropriate for opening the airway?

A. Head-tilt/chin-lift
B. Endotracheal intubation
C. Jaw thrust
D. Cricoid compression

63. You arrive at a home where a 7-year-old female who has been ill for the past five days with coughing, difficulty breathing, fever, and weakness suddenly loses consciousness. You find the patient lying supine on the living room floor with agonal breathing. Her limbs are cold, and her heart rate is 56 bpm. What should you do?

A. Administer rescue breaths with head-tilt/chin-lift at a rate of 20 to 30 per minute.
B. Commence chest compressions at a rate of 30 to two rescue breaths; apply AED pads if available.
C. Intubate the patient immediately and oxygenate with BVM.
D. Administer IV or IO epinephrine.

64. A 19-year-old male presents with difficulty breathing, wheezing, and swelling of the tongue. He has hives on his skin and a history of allergy to shellfish. Pulse is 108 bpm, and blood pressure is 90/60 mmHg. What is the most likely cause of this clinical state?

A. Anaphylaxis
B. Acute asthma exacerbation
C. Epiglottitis
D. Foreign body aspiration

65. A 45-year-old female presents with dyspnea of sudden onset. She is dehydrated. Her pulse is 60 bpm. Blood pressure is 80/40 mmHg. A paradoxical pulse; distended neck veins; and cold, clammy extremities are noted. The woman has a history of recurrent tuberculosis infection; on auscultation, heart sounds are muffled. What may be the possible cause of the woman's symptoms?

A. Pleural effusion
B. Cardiac tamponade
C. Heart failure
D. None of the above

66. A 15-year-old female in respiratory failure requires artificial ventilation. The signs of respiratory failure include all except which of the following?

A. Increased work of breathing
B. Poor chest wall movement
C. Cyanosis
D. Patient lying in a supine position

67. A 30-year-old male was found unconscious and unresponsive. His respirations are inefficient and require BVM ventilation. To open the airway, what should you do?

A. Jaw-thrust maneuver
B. Chin lift
C. Head-lift/chin sweep
D. Log-rolling

68. Your patient has difficulty breathing and chest tightness. You commence ventilation with a non-rebreather mask. What percentage of oxygen does a patient get from the non-rebreather mask?

A. 100%
B. 90%
C. 80%
D. 75%

69. While you are resuscitating an unconscious patient, he vomits copiously. These secretions cannot be removed quickly by suctioning. What should you do?

A. Sit the patient upright.
B. Log roll the patient to the side.
C. Give the patient high-flow oxygen using a non-rebreather mask.
D. Quickly arrange for transportation.

70. A 50-year-old male is apneic; he has occasional gasping breath with strange vocalizations. What type of respiration is this?

A. Agonal respiration
B. Cheyne-Stokes respiration
C. Hyperventilation
D. None of the above

71. You are delivering artificial ventilation to a 20-year-old male who was involved in a car crash. He is cyanosed with SPO2 90%. How do you know if ventilation is adequate?

A. Skin color improves
B. Chest rises and falls with ventilation
C. SaO2 increases to 92%
D. All of the above

72. A 45-year-old hypertensive male who suffered a stroke is lethargic and responsive to painful stimuli. You notice snoring respirations. When you insert a nasopharyngeal airway into the left nostril, you meet resistance. What should you do?

A. Force the nasopharyngeal airway in.
B. Try the other nostril.
C. Insert an oropharyngeal airway.
D. Select a smaller nasopharyngeal airway.

73. A 30-year-old pregnant female eating in a restaurant suddenly collapses. Her face turns blue, she is making choking sounds, and she is unable to breathe. What is the appropriate intervention?

A. Perform the Heimlich maneuver.
B. Commence chest thrusts.
C. Give rapid back blows.
D. Give high-flow oxygen with a non-rebreather mask.

74. You are called to attend to a 60-year-old patient with COPD. He is dyspneic, cyanosed, in a tripod position, and wheezing. What does *wheezing* mean?

A. The whistling sound heard during inspiration
B. The high-pitched sound heard on expiration
C. The low-pitched sound heard on auscultation
D. The high-pitched sound heard on expiration

75. Which of the following patients requires high Fowler's positioning?

A. An elderly female with orthopnea, blood-tinged sputum, and crackles in the lung bases
B. A young man with productive cough, fever, chest pain, and tachypnea
C. An elderly male who presents with wheezing and chest tightness
D. An apneic 18-month-old

76. An elderly, unconscious patient is making snoring sounds while breathing. What is the most common cause of airway obstruction in this type of patient?

A. The tongue
B. Secretions
C. Emesis
D. Foreign body

77. A 20-year-old male is unconscious and apneic after an overdose of a narcotic drug. While giving rescue breaths using a BVM, you notice the man's oxygen saturation has further declined. What is the appropriate intervention?

A. Reposition the patient's head.
B. Remove the oral airway.
C. Enable the pop-off valve.
D. Commence chest compressions.

78. While performing a secondary assessment in a patient with difficulty breathing, how should you determine oxygen saturation?

A. Pulse oximetry
B. Capnography
C. CPAP
D. Spirometry

79. A 14-year-old asthmatic presents with shortness of breath. He is anxious, cyanosed, and wheezing. He is sweating, cannot speak in full sentences, and has been unable to respond to initial treatment and bronchodilators. What is the likely cause of his condition?

A. Status asthmaticus
B. Foreign body obstruction
C. Croup
D. Vocal cord dysfunction

80. A 65-year-old hypertensive complains of sudden onset of chest tightness that lasts more than 30 minutes and radiates medially to his left arm. He is diaphoretic and anxious, and he feels nauseous. His respiration is 28 bpm, SPO2 94%, pulse rate 60 bpm, and blood pressure 110/90 mmHg. His skin is cold and clammy. The patient had similar symptoms six months prior, for which sublingual nitroglycerin was prescribed. What is the most appropriate intervention?

A. Commence high-flow oxygen via a non-rebreather mask.
B. Assist in giving nitroglycerin.
C. Arrange for transport.
D. Place in the high Fowler's position.

81. You have a 20-year-old patient in respiratory distress. The patient is tachypneic and breathing with accessory muscles. Her skin is pale and dusky, and she is restless. You are unable to do a pulse oximeter reading. What is the appropriate intervention?

A. Withhold oxygen until a pulse oximeter reading is available.
B. Administer high-flow oxygen using a non-rebreather mask.
C. Encourage the patient to breathe into a paper bag.
D. Talk the patient through the episode of distress.

82. A 60-year-old truck driver was involved in a road traffic accident. On your arrival at the scene with your partner, the patient is unresponsive but withdraws from painful stimuli. His skin is cold and clammy, pulse rate 110 bpm, blood pressure 90/60 mmHg. The man is making gurgling sounds and has a large right parietal hematoma on the scalp and periorbital ecchymosis. On auscultation, breath sounds are absent in the left hemithorax. As the EMT dispatched to the scene, what should you do to secure the airway?

A. Perform a jaw thrust with cervical spine protection to open the airway.
B. Perform a head-tilt/chin-lift to open the airway.
C. Insert a nasopharyngeal airway.
D. Suction the oropharynx to open the airway.

83. A 20-year-old female is hysterical after receiving emotional news. She is anxious, breathing deeply and rapidly. She complains of feeling unable to catch her breath, numbness, tingling sensations in her hands and feet, and dizziness. Her respiratory rate is 40 bpm. SaO2 is 92%. Blood pressure is 100/70 mmHg. You verbally instruct the patient to slow her breathing; however, she is unable to stop breathing rapidly. What is the appropriate intervention?

A. Encourage the patient to breathe into a paper bag.
B. Give supplemental oxygen and provide transport.
C. Encourage the patient to lie on her left lateral side.
D. Advise the patient to try breathing exercises.

84. A 20-year-old asthmatic complains of productive cough, pleuritic chest pain, difficulty in breathing, fever, headaches, and fatigue. On examination, he is tachypneic and febrile. Rhonchi are heard in the lung bases. SaO2 is 92%. What is the appropriate intervention?

A. Place the patient in a comfortable position and give supplemental oxygen.
B. Administer nebulized salbutamol.
C. Give blow-by humidified oxygen.
D. Continuous positive airway pressure should be considered.

85. An 18-month-old child is apneic with no respiratory effort after taking drugs from an unidentified container. You commence BVM ventilation. Which of the following statements is incorrect about giving artificial ventilation to this patient using the BVM?

A. You should place the patient's head in a neutral position to open the airway.
B. Gastric distention is common in such patients.
C. The pop-off valve must be disabled before treatment is commenced.
D. You should hyperextend the patient's head.

86. An 11-month-old baby has fast breathing. There is a history of fever, cough, drooling, and anorexia two days before presentation. Which of the following is a danger sign in a baby with fast breathing?

A. Hypothermia
B. Audible stridor in a calm baby
C. Refusal to feed
D. All of the above

87. While delivering BVM ventilation to a 6-year-old apneic female, you notice her chest does not rise with each ventilation. What should you do?

A. Reposition the child's head.
B. Apply more ventilation pressure.
C. Create a tighter mask seal.
D. Hyperextend the child's neck.

88. A 2-year-old swallows a peanut. He suddenly starts coughing, is in respiratory distress, and has audible stridor. He is tachypneic, flaring his nostrils, and agitated. His respiratory rate is 36 bpm. SaO2 is 92%. This child most likely has which of the following?

A. Complete airway obstruction
B. Partial airway obstruction
C. Anaphylaxis
D. None of the above

89. You attend to a 56-year-old female who complains of vaginal bleeding. Her last menstrual period was five years ago. Which of the following is not a likely diagnosis?

A. Ectopic gestation
B. Postcoital bleeding
C. Cervical cancer
D. Endometritis

90. Which of the following is true of the phases of the menstrual cycle?

A. Proliferative – occurs in the last two weeks of the menstrual cycle
B. Proliferative – caused by estrogen in the uterine lining
C. Secretory – uterus secretes progesterone
D. Secretory – estrogen increases, and progesterone decreases if the egg is not fertilized

91. Acute renal failure refers to the rapid loss of kidney function. Which of the following is not a prerenal cause of ARF?

A. Hemorrhage
B. Persistent vomiting
C. Rhabdomyolysis
D. Myocardial infarction

92. You attend to a 5-month-old child with diarrhea who has been poorly managed at home. On examination, he is irritable and distressed. His temperature is 37.7° C. The boy's mother tells you he is refusing to feed and has not passed any urine today. Which of the following presenting symptoms is most alarming?

A. Poorly managed diarrhea
B. Temperature of 37.7° C
C. Refusing to feed
D. Not passing urine

93. You and your partner are dispatched to the residence of a 45-year-old male who complains of severe flank pain that radiates to the groin, nausea, and vomiting. He is being managed for renal stones and is due for a follow-up visit next week. What is the appropriate intervention?

A. Turn on the faucet and encourage the patient to void.
B. Keep the patient comfortable and transport him gently.
C. Administer the patient's analgesic medications.
D. Place the patient in the supine position.

94. An EMT is alerted to attend to a 12-year-old male with scrotal pain. The boy was playing football on a school playground when the ball was accidentally thrown at his scrotum. What is the most likely diagnosis?

A. Penile fracture
B. Epididymitis
C. Testicular torsion
D. None of the above

95. A 16-year-old male complains of progressively worsening scrotal pain, fever, and chills. He denies a history of trauma but admits to having unprotected sexual intercourse with multiple sexual partners. What is the most likely diagnosis?

A. Epididymitis
B. Testicular torsion
C. Priapism
D. Syphilis

96. Priapism is a persistent, often painful, penile erection that occurs for more than four hours without sexual stimulation. Which of the following is not a cause of this condition?

A. Sickle cell disease
B. Leukemia
C. Malaria
D. Chronic renal failure

97. Concerning urinary symptoms, which of the following definitions is incorrect?

A. Hematuria – passage of frank or microscopic blood in the urine
B. Frequency – involuntary leakage of urine from a full bladder
C. Strangury – slow, painful, unintentional passage of small volumes of urine
D. Nocturia – frequent nighttime urination

98. You are called to attend to a 72-year-old male. You find him lying in bed with a retaining catheter. He complains of weakness, fever, and chills for the last four days. On examination, his respiratory rate is 26 cpm, pulse is 110 bpm, and blood pressure is 90/70 mmHg. Which of the following is not an appropriate intervention?

A. Sitting the patient up
B. Commencing supplemental oxygen
C. Placing the patient in the supine position
D. Preparing to transport the patient

99. A 59-year-old female is being managed for chronic kidney disease. Which of the following will this patient be at risk of?

A. Recurrent infections
B. Anemia
C. Heart failure
D. All of the above

100. You and your partner are dispatched to the residence of a 16-year-old female who is seen clutching her abdomen while lying on a bed. She complains of generalized abdominal pain, nausea, and vomiting. On examination, she has a temperature of 37.6° C. RR 28 cpm, PR 107 bpm, and BP 90/70 mmHg. Which of the following interventions is inappropriate?

A. Encouraging the patient to eat some food
B. Placing the patient in the supine position
C. Administering oxygen
D. Maintaining body temperature

101. A 45-year-old female complains of severe right upper quadrant pain, which is sharp and radiates to the back. She ate a meal of pork about an hour ago. What is the most likely diagnosis?

A. Cholecystitis
B. Peptic ulcer disease
C. Pelvic inflammatory disease
D. Gastroenteritis

102. A 53-year-old male being managed for chronic liver disease vomits large amounts of frank blood. He was out with his friends last night and drank a lot of alcohol. On examination, he appears anxious with a pulse of 110 bpm and blood pressure of 90/63 mmHg. Which of the following is an appropriate intervention?

A. Lay the patient in the left lateral recumbent position.
B. Suction any blood in the patient's airway.
C. Maintain the patient's body temperature.
D. All of the above.

103. A 29-year-old cigarette smoker complains of a burning sensation just below his sternum. This pain is usually worse after meals, and he had lunch about two hours ago. The man also feels nauseous. What is his most likely diagnosis?

A. Peptic ulcer disease
B. Gastroenteritis
C. Mallory-Weiss tear
D. Cholecystitis

104. Peritonitis refers to irritation of the abdominal membranes by gastrointestinal contents that have leaked out into the abdominal cavity following a rupture. Which of the following statements is false concerning peritonitis?

A. It can cause very serious abdominal infections.
B. Transporting patients with flexed knees may help reduce pain.
C. It may be fatal if not properly and promptly managed.
D. None of the above.

105. You and your partner are dispatched to the home of a 53-year-old male who complains of abdominal pain that suddenly started 20 minutes ago. He now feels faint and nauseous. On examination, his respiratory rate is 28 cpm with a thready pulse of 115 bpm. Blood pressure of 85/63. You are unable to feel a femoral pulse. Which of the following best explains this scenario?

A. Cholecystitis
B. Pancreatitis
C. Peptic ulcer disease
D. Ruptured aortic abdominal aneurysm

106. A 15-year-old female complains of abdominal pain, vomiting, and passage of loose stools. Symptoms started shortly after she ate a sandwich. On examination, her vital signs are within normal limits. What condition best fits this description?

A. Gastroenteritis
B. Cholecystitis
C. Pelvic inflammatory disease
D. Appendicitis

107. Upper GI bleeding may present as the passage of dark-colored stool or as vomiting of frank blood. Which of the following is not a cause of upper GI bleeding?

A. Peptic ulcer disease
B. Mallory-Weiss tear
C. Gastritis
D. Diverticular disease

108. An ectopic pregnancy refers to the implantation of a zygote in a location other than the uterine cavity. Which of the following statements is false concerning an ectopic pregnancy?

A. Abdominal pain may be absent.
B. A pregnancy test must be positive.
C. There may be no history of a missed period.
D. The majority of ectopic pregnancies occur in the fallopian tubes.

109. You are attending to a 23-year-old female with a first-trimester pregnancy who is experiencing cramping lower abdominal pain, vaginal bleeding, and passage of fetal parts through her vagina. Emergency management of this patient will include all except which of the following?

A. Providing high-concentration oxygen
B. Providing emotional support
C. Transporting any fetal tissues expelled to the hospital
D. Transporting the patient in the high Fowler's position

110. You and your partner are dispatched to the residence of a 20-year-old primigravida at 26 weeks gestation who complains of epigastric pain, nausea, and vomiting. You notice she has facial and limb swelling, and her blood pressure is 149/94 mmHg. Urinalysis – ++ of protein. The patient was normotensive before this pregnancy. What is your most likely diagnosis?

A. Eclampsia
B. Preeclampsia
C. Chronic hypertension
D. Peptic ulcer disease

111. Which of the following is false concerning the management of a person with eclampsia?

A. The patient may require high-concentration oxygen.
B. You should reduce light in the patient compartment.
C. You should transport the patient in the left lateral recumbent position.
D. You should allow ambulation.

112. You receive a distress call from a 42-year-old female, G5P4 at 32 weeks gestation, who complains of a sharp abdominal pain of sudden onset and vaginal bleeding. On examination, she has a rigid, tender uterus. Respiratory rate is 28 breaths per minute, pulse of 100 bpm, and blood pressure of 90/60 mmHg. Which of the following conditions is the woman likely suffering from?

A. Abruptio placenta
B. Missed abortion
C. Placenta previa
D. Spontaneous abortion

113. A 32-year-old G2P1 with one previous caesarean section complains of painless vaginal bleeding. Following your assessment, you suspect a diagnosis of placenta previa. Which of the following steps is not an appropriate intervention?

A. Administering high-concentration oxygen
B. Treating hypovolemia
C. Packing the birth canal with absorbent material
D. Transporting the patient in the left lateral recumbent position

114. Uterine rupture is an obstetric emergency. Which of the following scenarios is at the least risk of a rupture?

A. A 42-year-old G5P4 with two previous caesarean sections
B. A G3P2 with prolonged obstructed labor
C. A 32-year-old G2P1 with blunt abdominal trauma
D. A 35-year-old P2 with severe abdominal pain who was involved in a road traffic accident

115. Which of the following is false concerning emergency childbirth outside a hospital setting?

A. For a competent emergency responder, contacting medical direction for the decision to commit to delivery is not necessary.
B. Body substance isolation/personal protective equipment must be used.
C. Oxygen and resuscitation equipment for both mother and baby should be available.
D. Post-delivery, the placenta should be wrapped and transported to the hospital along with the mother and baby.

116. Concerning pediatric circulation, which of the following is false?

A. Children compensate effectively in shock but decompensate rapidly.
B. Blood pressure is a reliable indicator of perfusion in a pediatric patient.
C. Mental status change is a good indicator of hypoperfusion.
D. Bradycardia is a late sign of low oxygen.

117. In using a traction splint in a patient with a femoral fracture, what procedures should not be observed?

A. Applying a splint above the injured thigh
B. Manually stabilizing the injured thigh
C. Applying mechanical traction
D. Applying proximal and distal securing devices

118. You are called to attend to a 55-year-old female with chills and rigors. On examination, you observe a weak pulse and suspected hypothermia. Which of the following terms is incorrect about how heat loss occurs?

A. Radiation
B. Conduction
C. Evaporation
D. Effervescence

119. In assessing the above patient, what is the least likely question you should ask in assessing severity and protocol of management?

A. How is the patient's environment?
B. What is the patient's influence on the environment?
C. Does the patient have any history of loss of consciousness?
D. What is the source of the hypothermia?

120. Which of the following is the most practical way of protecting yourself from infections?

A. Sterile gloves
B. Handwashing
C. Eye goggles
D. Sizing up a scene

Test 4: Answers and Explanations

1. (B) An adult male with an open fracture to the thigh, cool and clammy skin, radial pulse absent, RR 30 cpm.
This patient should be tagged red and given immediate care. Patient A and D are tagged yellow (delayed), and Patient C is tagged black (dead).

2. (A) RR less than 30 cpm
This is not a feature of red-tag patients. Patients in this category require immediate treatment. Their cardiopulmonary function is compromised, and they are likely to die if they are not stabilized.

3. (A) Circulation is assessed first.
This statement is false because in START triage, respiration is assessed first, followed by circulation, then mental status.

4. (C) Start from where you are.
After relocating the walking wounded to another area, you should start triaging from where you are and move in an organized manner. Keep tabs on the number of casualties.

5. (D) OSHA
The Occupational Safety and Health Administration (OSHA) is focused on providing a healthy and safe working environment for all workers in the United States. It is not a resource for confirming hazardous materials. Such resources include DOT placards, UN numbers, North American Response Guide (NARG), shipping papers, material safety data sheets (MSDS), and the National Fire Protection Agency (NFPA) placard system.

6. (B) Access with Level A PPE is required.
This statement is correct. The hot zone is the area of immediate release of contaminants. The risk of primary contamination is very high. Therefore, access is given only to highly trained personnel dressed in Level A PPE, which has a contained self-breathing apparatus.

7. (C) The PPE must contain air-purifying respirators.
This statement is correct. The warm zone is the area of decontamination. Because the risk of secondary contamination is high, all personnel must wear Level B PPE with air-purifying respirators. This zone is assessed by health personnel responsible for managing and triaging victims.

8. (B) There is a risk of secondary contamination.
This statement is correct. The cold zone is also called the clean zone. A good example is ER units. Although standard precautions can protect personnel from secondary contamination, contaminated patients can erroneously enter the cold zone.

9. (A) Gases are common sources of secondary contamination.
This statement is false because gas particles rarely cause secondary contamination. Most implicated substances are liquids and particles.

10. (A) Neutralization
In neutralization, a substance is given to neutralize the effects of the contaminant. This mode is rarely used because it takes time to find the appropriate neutralizing material and there is a huge risk of the formation of an exothermic reaction.

11. (D) Urinary retention
You should not expect patients to demonstrate urinary retention in this scenario. Nerve agents inhibit acetylcholinesterase, an enzyme that metabolizes acetylcholine. The prolonged action of acetylcholine on muscarinic and nicotinic receptors causes parasympathetic hyperactivity. Symptoms include rhinorrhea, miosis, bronchoconstriction, twitching, sweating, muscle fasciculations, urinary incontinence, diarrhea, salivation, abdominal cramps, vomiting, and seizures. Death is caused by apnea from bronchospasms.

12. (A) Park your vehicle at a safe distance.
The most appropriate response is to park your vehicle at a safe distance and assess the scene with a pair of binoculars. Next, call for assistance from a trained hazmat response team.

13. (D) Diarrhea
Mustard gas does not cause diarrhea. It is a vesicant agent that causes erythema and blisters on the skin. It also causes redness; tearing; swelling of the cornea; and conjunctival and respiratory symptoms, like cough, wheezing, stridor, hoarseness, and laryngospasms.

14. (D) Cellular anoxia
Hydrogen sulfide and cyanides are both asphyxiants. At the cellular level, they prevent oxidative phosphorylation. This causes cellular anoxia because the body's tissues are unable to extract oxygen from the red blood cells. Symptoms of cellular anoxia include conjunctivitis, headaches, confusion, chest pain, hyperventilation, vomiting, and ataxia.

15. (C) It gives a high level of respiratory protection.
This statement is correct. Level B PPE gives a high level of respiratory protection. However, the level of skin and eye protection is not as high as Level A. This is because Level A PPE is made with chemical-resistant material that is splash resistant.

16. (D) D
Level D protection provides the lowest form of protection. An example is the uniform worn by firefighters.

17. (C) It is caused by spores from aerobic bacteria.
This statement is false because anthrax is caused by spores from anaerobic bacteria.

18. (C) Aerosols
Aerosols are the most common route of dissemination of a biological weapon. Biological agents are readily disseminated as aerosols because aerosols are nonvolatile and lack characteristic smells.

19. (B) Tetanus toxin
Tetanus is not considered a threat by the CDC. Although there are over 100 identified toxins, only 4 toxins are classified as high-threat agents by the CDC: botulinum toxin, ricin toxin, epsilon toxin, and staphylococcus enterotoxin B.

20. (A) Excessive salivation
You should not expect to see excessive salivation in this scenario, as botulinum toxin causes dryness of the oral cavity. Other symptoms include slurred speech, drooping eyelids, dysphagia, double vision, and absent pulmonary light reflex.

21. (D) Small surface area compared to the overall size
This is not a possible predisposing factor in this scenario. Pediatric patients are more predisposed to hypothermia than adults because of their large surface area compared to their overall size. This factor, along with cold environments and immersion, increases the risk of hypothermia in children.

22. (C) Well-developed ability to shiver during cold
Children and infants do not have a well-developed ability to shiver. This predisposes them to hypothermia. Small body mass and less fat reduce their ability to save heat within the body.

23. (C) Chronic cough
Conditions that can increase this patient's risk for shock are hypovolemia, hypoperfusion, and hyperglycemia. Chronic cough can worsen this patient's respiratory function but not her circulatory function.

24. (D) Low blood pressure
Low blood pressure is the least likely symptom you should look out for during your examination. If the patient has hypotension, he may experience dizziness, syncope, and altered sensorium.

25. (A) Joint pain
Joint pain is the least likely sign you expect to see in this patient. The signs that can be elicited in this patient are cyanosis, blanching, pallor, poor coordination, etc.

26. (A) If the patient is unresponsive, massage his extremities.
If a patient is not responding appropriately, you should not massage his extremities. The patient may be at risk of deep vein thrombosis, and massaging may dislodge clots and trigger a pulmonary embolism. Also, avoid putting any food or drink through the mouth to avoid aspiration and chemical pneumonitis.

27. (D) Restrict oral intake even if the patient can tolerate it.
This statement is incorrect. If the patient is alert, responsive, and able to tolerate food and drink, oral feeding should be allowed with close observation and monitoring. The aim is to increase the patient's body temperature to restore body metabolic functions. Food restriction is necessary for unconscious and unstable patients, since they are at risk of aspiration.

28. (C) Blisters
You are unlikely to see blisters on this patient, as they are not early features of localized cold injuries. Common signs are blanching with pale-blue discoloration, inflammation, and numbness.

29. (B) Tingling sensation
A tingling sensation may be present only in an early and superficial cold injury and if the injury is rewarmed. The skin in a late and deep injury may also be white, waxy, and sometimes cyanotic. Blisters are usually painful late features of cold injuries. Swelling is seen in both the early and late stages of an injury. There can also be tenderness and other signs of an inflammatory response to injury.

30. (D) You should massage or rub the injury.
Massaging or rubbing of injured extremities is contraindicated, as this may worsen the state. Hyperbaric oxygen is recommended to improve the patient's response. Replacing all wet or cold clothing with warm and dry clothes is the first essential step, as patients may be at risk of hypothermia.

31. (A) Low relative humidity in children
Low relative humidity only increases the body's ability to release or lose heat through evaporation. This does not result in heat injury. High relative humidity can increase the risk of heat injury. The poor thermoregulatory activity in infants predisposes them to frequent fluctuations in body temperature regulation. And unlike adults, infants need to be changed by a caregiver.

32. (A) Bradycardia
Patients with intensive heat injuries are unlikely to present with bradycardia. Such patients' heart rates are rapid due to increased cardiac output. Tachycardia may be accompanied by nausea and dyspnea. Blood pressure is low with generalized weakness and exhaustion. In addition, disorientation, fainting spells, and, in extreme cases, loss of consciousness may be present.

33. (B) Left lateral position
For unconscious or unresponsive patients, a left lateral position is appropriate to reduce the risk of aspiration of vomitus from the esophagus into the trachea. This position also prevents the tongue from falling backward and restricting airflow and airway patency.

34. (C) 30% to 40%
The incidence of tissue damage from cat bites is limited compared to dogs. However, cats have a 30% to 40% higher risk of infections. Also, cat bites inflict deeper puncture wounds that penetrate even to the tendons and bones. The infection rate for dog bite injuries is 15% to 20%.

35. (C) Human
The human mouth harbors a large number of harmful microorganisms, making human bites the most infectious of all bites.

36. (D) Cat-scratch disease is life threatening.
This statement is untrue. Cat-scratch disease, caused by Bartonella henselae, is not a life-threatening disease, though it is usually unpleasant.

37. (A) Tissue necrosis
This is not a symptom of a bite from a black widow spider. Tissue necrosis, or necrotic arachnidism, is a key feature of a bite from the brown recluse spider.

38. (C) Venomous bites by pit vipers cause swelling after an hour.
This statement is incorrect. Swelling or inflammation at the site of injury usually starts about 10 minutes after a bite. There is also skin discoloration and blisters. Muscle contractions, rapid breathing, and elevated heart rate are common results of severe poisoning. The occasional inability to envenomate their prey does not rule out the fact that pit vipers are venomous snakes.
39. (D) If the stinger is still present, you should scrape it out with forceps.
This response is inappropriate in the management of this patient. Using forceps or any similar object to hold the stinger of a snakebite may cause possible squeezing of the venom sac of the stinger into the tissue, thus worsening the patient's condition.

40. (D) Deferred access
Deferred access is not part of the chain of survival for successful resuscitation. Early access is essential for successful resuscitation, according to the AHA.

41. (A) Lay the woman in a supine position, administer oxygen by intranasal cannula, perform an ECG, and quickly transport the patient to the hospital.
Because of the hypotension, laying the woman on her back will reduce cardiac workload. Supplemental oxygen will help her respiration.

42. (A) Place the patient in a supine position and commence supplemental oxygen.
This is the appropriate intervention. The supine position will be best for this patient on account of her hypotension.

43. (C) Aortic aneurysm
An aortic aneurysm is the most likely cause of this presentation. It can present with unequal pulses in arms or legs.

44. (B) Anaphylaxis
Anaphylaxis is least likely to cause chest pain. It is an exaggerated immune response and may present with hives, swelling of the upper airway, and hypotension but rarely chest pain.

45. (A) Begin CPR with ventilation, not compressions.
This is not important for high-quality CPR. CPR should begin with chest compressions.
46. (B) Lay the man in a supine position, assess his saturation, and give supplemental oxygen if needed.

This is the most appropriate intervention. Sepsis can result from an untreated or poorly treated UTI. In this situation, laying the patient in the supine position gives the heart less work. Also, saturating with oxygen will ensure that the tissues are perfused with oxygen.

47. (C) Pulmonary edema in cardiogenic shock
This is the most likely cause of the woman's difficulty breathing. The crackles heard on auscultation indicate fluid in the lungs. This will most likely be seen in cardiogenic shock.

48. (A) Hypotension
Hypotension is a side effect commonly seen with nitroglycerin use. The drug is not administered to patients with systolic pressures of less than 100 mmHg.

49. (D) Furosemide
This medication is not used by EMTs in cardiovascular emergencies. Furosemide is a diuretic used in the treatment of hypertension but is not effective in emergencies.

50. (B) Stage 2
Stage 2 of hypovolemia is when 15% to 30% of total blood is lost (less than three pints).

51. (C) Vomiting
Vomiting can be caused by increased intracranial pressure but rarely ever by reduced cerebral blood flow.

52. (B) Dehydration
This patient is most likely dehydrated from the continuous vomiting and subsequent reduction of his body fluid volume.

53. (A) Anaphylaxis
Anaphylactic reactions to latex are common and can present as described.

54. (B) Cold-water immersion
This is the most effective treatment for exertional heatstroke in the field.

55. (A) Myocardial infarction
This patient has risk factors for myocardial infarction and symptoms that point toward MI.

56. (A) Two inches
Compressions should be done at a depth of two inches.

57. (C) Three
A maximum of three shocks can be given if a shockable rhythm is still detected by the AED after previous shocks.

58. (B) 10 seconds
You should spend about 10 seconds or less when assessing breathing and pulse. If these are absent, CPR should be started immediately.

59. (C) Place the man in the cardiac position and administer supplemental oxygen.
This patient most likely has pulmonary edema from cardiogenic shock. Placing him in a supine position will make breathing difficult, but lifting the head of the bed will provide some relief. Supplemental oxygen can be given.

60. (C) Neurogenic
Neurogenic shock usually occurs following trauma to the cervical spine, causing loss of sympathetic tone and decreasing the systemic vascular resistance.

61. (B) Perform a rhythm check every 10 minutes, lasting no more than 10 seconds. This is not one of the five main components of high-quality CPR. Also, a rhythm check should be done every 2 minutes, lasting no more than 10 seconds.

62. (C) Jaw thrust
This is the most appropriate intervention in this scenario. You should suspect a possible cervical injury from the history obtained, so a jaw thrust will theoretically limit cervical motion.

63. (A) Administer rescue breaths with head-tilt/chin-lift at a rate of 20 to 30 per minute.
This intervention is most appropriate. According to the algorithm, in a patient with abnormal breathing but a palpable pulse, rescue breathing is the recommended intervention at a rate of 20 to 30 breaths per minute.

64. (A) Anaphylaxis

The case scenario shows the presence of hives, tongue swelling, and hypotension. This is indicative of anaphylaxis. Acute asthma exacerbation will not cause tongue swelling; epiglottitis will likely present with fever and upper respiratory symptoms such as drooling; and foreign body aspiration is unlikely.

65. (B) Cardiac tamponade

A medical history of tuberculosis infection with increased jugular venous pressure, muffled heart sounds, pulsus paradoxus, and shock are strongly suggestive of cardiac tamponade. Pleural effusion and heart failure may cause muffling of heart sounds; however, a paradoxical pulse is unlikely.

66. (D) Patient lying in a supine position

This is not a symptom of respiratory failure. Patients with respiratory failure are unable to lie down or lean back. Most maintain the tripod position. Increased work of breathing, cyanosis, and poor chest wall expansion point to respiratory failure.

67. (A) Jaw-thrust maneuver

A jaw thrust should be used to open a patient's airway when the mechanism of injury is not known. Head lift, log rolling, and head-lift/chin sweep are not correct maneuvers to be used on this patient.

68. (B) 90%

A non-rebreather can deliver up to 90% oxygen. It is indicated in patients who are breathing adequately but show signs of hypoxia.

69. (B) Log roll the patient to the side.

The patient should be log rolled if secretions cannot be cleared by suctioning. Options A, C, and D are not appropriate.

70. (A) Agonal respiration

Agonal respirations are occasional gasping breaths, labored breathing, and strange vocalizations that may be seen just before death. Cheyne-Stokes and hyperventilation are not associated with gasping breaths.

71. (D) All of the above

Good chest rise, skin color improvement, heart rate returning to normal, and improving oxygen saturation all indicate adequate ventilation.

72. (B) Try the other nostril.
If the airway cannot be inserted into one nostril, you should try the other nostril. Never force the airway adjunct into the nostril. An oropharyngeal airway will cause gagging, as the patient is responsive to verbal stimuli. A properly sized airway should always be used.

73. (B) Commence chest thrusts.
Chest thrusts are given for pregnant or obese victims to relieve obstruction. The Heimlich maneuver and back blows are inappropriate for this patient. A non-rebreather mask is not indicated for a patient with ongoing airway obstruction.

74. (A) The whistling sound heard during inspiration
Wheezing is a whistling sound heard on inspiration and/or expiration.

75. (A) An elderly female with orthopnea, blood-tinged sputum, and crackles in the lung bases
This is a typical presentation of pulmonary edema, which is an indication for high Fowler's positioning in this patient. Wheezing and chest tightness, productive cough, and apneic patients do not require high Fowler's positioning.

76. (A) The tongue
The tongue is the most common cause of airway obstruction in an unconscious patient. This is because the tongue has a reduced muscle tone, which can cause it to relax and fall backward, blocking the airway. To prevent this, an oropharyngeal airway should be inserted. Secretions, emesis, and foreign bodies are less likely to cause an airway obstruction in this patient.

77. (A) Reposition the patient's head.
Desaturation shows respiration is inadequate. Repositioning the patient's head using a jaw thrust or chin lift will open up the airway and improve saturation on subsequent attempts at ventilation. Removing the oral airway, enabling a pop-off valve, and administering chest compressions will not enable adequate ventilation or improve the patient's level of oxygen saturation.

78. (A) Pulse oximetry
Pulse oximetry determines how well a patient is being oxygenated. It measures the transmission of red and near-infrared light through the arterial bed. Capnography determines carbon dioxide concentration in exhaled air. Continuous positive airway pressure helps improve alveolar ventilation, and spirometry helps assess lung function.

79. (A) Status asthmaticus
Status asthmaticus is a likely cause. Acute asthma is not responsive to initial treatment and bronchodilators. Foreign body obstruction will cause stridor; croup will present with drooling and audible stridor; and vocal cord dysfunction causes wheezing on inspiration.

80. (B) Assist in giving nitroglycerin.
This should be the first-line treatment in acute myocardial infarction, as indicated. You can give oxygen and arrange for transport thereafter. The high Fowler's position is not indicated in this case scenario.

81. (B) Administer high-flow oxygen using a non-rebreather mask.
This is the appropriate intervention. Oxygen should never be withheld from a patient when there is respiratory distress and evidence of hypoxia. Breathing into a paper bag will cause the woman to retain CO_2, and talking her through the episode will not improve her immediate condition.

82. (A) Perform a jaw thrust with cervical spine protection to open the airway.
You should always maintain cervical spine immobilization. Perform a jaw thrust to open the airway. The nasopharyngeal airway should be avoided in case of a suspected basilar skull fracture. A head-tilt/chin-lift is contraindicated in cases of suspected neck injury or cervical spine injury. Suctioning can be done to clear the airway of blood and secretions. However, the spine has to be stabilized and protected, and the airway must be opened using a jaw thrust before suction can be applied.

83. (B) Give supplemental oxygen and provide transport.
This scenario depicts hyperventilation syndrome. In the management of hyperventilation syndrome, you should reassure the patient and verbally instruct her to slow her breathing. If that does not work, give supplemental oxygen and provide transport to emergency care. Breathing into a paper bag is no longer advised. Lying on the left lateral side will not improve the patient's symptoms, and advising breathing exercises alone is inadequate at this level of care.

84. (A) Place the patient in a comfortable position and give supplemental oxygen.
This is the appropriate intervention. The patient has pneumonia with reduced oxygen saturation. Oxygen is needed in this patient. Nebulized salbutamol, blow-by humidified oxygen, and CPAP will not be of any benefit to him.

85. (D) You should hyperextend the patient's head.
This statement is incorrect. While using a BVM to ventilate an infant, the head should be placed in the correct neutral position. You should avoid hyperextension of the head and excess bag pressure. Ventilate until adequate chest rise. Gastric distention is more common in children, and the pop-off valve must be disabled to ensure adequate ventilation.

86. (D) All of the above
Hypothermia, audible stridor in a calm baby, and refusal to feed are danger signs in a baby with fast breathing. Other signs include cyanosis, lethargy, chest retractions, and convulsions.

87. (A) Reposition the child's head.
Repositioning the child's head will open up the airway and allow adequate ventilation. Applying more ventilation pressure will only cause gastric distention. Create a tighter mask seal only if the air is escaping from the mask and hyperextending the neck will occlude the airway.

88. (B) Partial airway obstruction
The child is coughing and has audible stridor, which indicates that air can pass through the level of obstruction. If he had a complete obstruction, he would not be able to make a sound. Cyanosis may be present, and the child may exhibit choking signs. Anaphylaxis is unlikely because it presents with hives, hypotension, reddening of the oropharynx, and drooling.

89. (A) Ectopic gestation.
Although this can present with vaginal bleeding, ectopic gestation is an unlikely cause of vaginal bleeding in this post-menopausal woman.
90. (B) Proliferative – caused by estrogen in the uterine lining
The proliferative phase of the menstrual cycle occurs in the first two weeks and is caused by estrogen, which increases the proliferation of the uterine lining. In the secretory phase, there is increased progesterone production by the luteal cells of the ovary. Estrogen production is reduced if the egg is not fertilized.

91. (C) Rhabdomyolysis
Rhabdomyolysis is not a prerenal cause of ARF. Myoglobin released from muscle tissues as they break down causes direct injury to renal cells. Rhabdomyolysis is therefore a cause of intrinsic renal damage.

92. (D) Not passing urine
All the presenting symptoms are significant; however, the presence of anuria indicates renal failure. Urgent intervention is needed.

93. (B) Keep the patient comfortable and transport him gently.
There is not much an EMT can do to alleviate this patient's pain and discomfort. He should be kept in the most comfortable position and transported as gently as possible.

94. (C) Testicular torsion
Testicular torsion is the most likely diagnosis. This is the twisting of the spermatic cord, leading to ischemia of the testicles and surrounding structures. Risk factors include cold temperatures, physical activity, and scrotal trauma. It is most common between ages 12 and 16.

95. (A) Epididymitis
Epididymitis is the most likely diagnosis. This is the inflammation of the epididymis, a coiled, tubular structure posterior to the testes where sperm is stored and matures. It may be caused by sexually transmitted infections, urinary tract infections, and some medications.

96. (D) Chronic renal failure
Chronic renal failure is not a cause of priapism. Causes of priapism include injury/trauma to the penis/perineum, spinal cord injury, and a foreign body lodged in the genitourinary tract.

97. (B) Frequency – involuntary leakage of urine from a full bladder
Urinary frequency is the need to urinate many times during the day but in normal or less than normal volume. It is different from urge incontinence (the involuntary leakage of urine from a full bladder) or polyuria (passage of more than three liters of urine in a day).

98. (A) Sitting the patient up
Placing the patient in a sitting position will lower his blood pressure and be detrimental to his condition. The presentation of this patient is suggestive of shock secondary to a likely urinary infection.

99. (D) All of the above
Chronic kidney disease affects all systems of the body and may cause recurrent infection, anemia, and heart failure. Patients should be encouraged to adhere to therapy as much as possible and report any problems.

100. (A) Encouraging the patient to eat some food
A patient with an acute abdomen should not be given oral foods or medications.

101. (A) Cholecystitis
Cholecystitis is the most likely diagnosis. This refers to gall bladder inflammation often caused by gallstones. Other symptoms include nausea, vomiting, and indigestion. This patient should be placed in a comfortable position and transported. Avoid giving anything by mouth.

102. (D) All of the above.
You should lay the patient in the left lateral recumbent position, suction any blood in the patient's airway, and maintain the patient's body temperature. This patient will also require high-flow oxygen via a non-rebreather mask and rapid transportation.

103. (A) Peptic ulcer disease
A peptic ulcer is the most likely diagnosis. This refers to small erosions of the gastric or duodenal lining. Patients usually experience a burning or gnawing discomfort in the upper abdomen or back. There may be bleeding, resulting in hematemesis and/or melena.

104. (D) None of the above.
None of these statements are false. It is true that peritonitis can cause very serious abdominal infections. Transporting patients with flexed knees may help reduce pain. The condition may be fatal if not properly and promptly managed. Patients may have fever, nausea, vomiting, and, in severe cases, shock.

105. (D) Ruptured aortic abdominal aneurysm
A ruptured aortic aneurysm best explains this scenario. This is a life-threatening condition. The patient should be managed per shock protocol and transported to a hospital as quickly and gently as possible.

106. (A) Gastroenteritis
Gastroenteritis is the infection of the gastrointestinal tract by bacteria or viruses. It is caused by ingestion of contaminated food or water. It may also cause dehydration and, in more severe cases, shock.

107. (D) Diverticular disease
Diverticular disease is not a cause of upper GI bleeding. It is a cause of lower GI bleeding and refers to outpouchings on the walls of the large intestine. Other symptoms include abdominal pain, nausea, and change in bowel habits.

108. (B) A pregnancy test must be positive.
This statement is false concerning an ectopic pregnancy. Depending on the gestational age of the fetus, serum B-HCG may not be high enough to be assayed, especially if a urine sample is used; thus, a pregnancy test may be negative in these patients.

109. (D) Transporting the patient in the high Fowler's position
This should not be part of this patient's emergency management. The patient should be transported gently in the Trendelenburg position. In this position, the body is laid supine at a 15- to 30-degree incline with the feet raised above the head. This position increases venous return to the heart.

110. (B) Preeclampsia
Preeclampsia is the most likely diagnosis. This refers to hypertension, proteinuria, and edema that occurs in the second half of pregnancy in a previously normotensive, non-proteinuric woman. It usually occurs with first pregnancies and can progress to eclampsia or other complications if not promptly managed.

111. (D) You should allow ambulation.
This statement is false. In a patient with eclampsia, excessive stimulation (including ambulation) should be avoided as much as possible. She should be gently transported to a hospital in the left lateral recumbent position.

112. (A) Abruptio placenta
Abruptio placenta should be suspected in older, hypertensive and/or multigravid patients who present with abdominal pain and mild to moderate vaginal bleeding. Until proven otherwise, third-trimester abdominal pain equals abruptio placenta.

113. (C) Packing the birth canal with absorbent material
This step is not an appropriate intervention. Any attempts to arrest bleeding by packing the birth canal may only precipitate further hemorrhage. At best, a vulval pad should be put in place to collect the blood while the patient is transported as quickly as possible to the hospital.

114. (D) A 35-year-old P2 with severe abdominal pain who was involved in a road traffic accident
This scenario describes a nonpregnant female; hence, trauma to other abdominal viscera is more likely from a road traffic accident.

115. (A) For a competent emergency responder, contacting medical direction for the decision to commit to delivery is not necessary.
This statement is false. If delivery is imminent, EMTs should always contact medical direction for a decision to commit to delivery. Medical direction should be contacted again for permission to transport if delivery does not occur within 10 minutes.

116. (B) Blood pressure is a reliable indicator of perfusion in a pediatric patient.
This statement is false. Blood pressure is usually an unreliable indicator of perfusion in this age group. When hypoperfusion sets in, children can maintain adequate blood pressure for longer times than adults, but they decompensate faster.

117. (A) Applying a splint above the injured thigh
This procedure should not be performed. The splint should be applied under the injured region and secured with support straps to a longboard. This is to prevent the movement of splints. After applying the proximal securing device (ischial strap) and distal securing device (ankle hitch), reevaluate them to ensure they are intact. Manual mechanical traction is needed when using a bipolar traction splint. Reassessment of the pulse and sensation of limb tissue distal to the focus of injury is necessary.

118. (D) Effervescence
This term is incorrect about how heat loss occurs. Hypothermia in humans can occur from radiation, conduction, and evaporation. Effervescence refers to the escape of gas from an aqueous solution and the resultant fizzing that occurs. A common example is the opening of carbonated drinks and beer.

119. (B) What is the patient's influence on the environment?
The patient's influence on the environment is of little importance in ascertaining severity and management and plays no role in the management of this patient. The patient's environment, the source of hypothermia, and any history of loss of consciousness after the injury and their effects on the patient are key in assessing severity and helping management.

120. (B) Handwashing
Handwashing is the most practical way of protecting yourself from infections. Always wash your hands after handling patients.

Made in the USA
Las Vegas, NV
17 March 2022